"This book is an extraordinary and valuable source of information about natural healing fundamentals for maintaining good health and wellbeing. It reveals endured wisdoms and secrets more than five thousand years old. I personally benefited from using exercises and nutritional information that were explicitly described in the book—I retired from office at age eighty-eight. Although the target is dementia and aging, the information applies to all aspects of remaining fit and healthy. It is detailed, shares actual cases, easy to understand, and the exercise illustrations are precise. I urgently recommend this book to people of all ages who want to stay healthy."

*—U.S. Senator Daniel K. Akaka (RET)*

"As the average human life span has steadily increased since the last century, dementia has become a major challenge to the wellbeing of the aging population. How to prevent, treat and improve dementia is a task our society faces. To solve this task, a combined effort is needed from different philosophies and medical fields—a place where the East meets the West. Stephen Rath has studied with Grandmaster for many years, and observed numerous successes of Grandmaster's Qigong exercises in helping people with dementia. This book provides clear and concise information about Traditional Chinese Medicine (TCM) and Western Medicine in order to help readers understand Qigong's benefit for this illness. The format of the exercises are easy to understand and practice. I hope this book will bring new light in fighting dementia and improving the quality of life for our elders."

*—Dr. Shi Cheng, MM (China), Dipl. Ac., Vice President and Co-Founder of*
*Colorado School of Traditional Chinese Medicine (CSTCM), Denver, CO*

*of related interest*

**Chair Yoga**
Seated Exercises for Health and Wellbeing
*Edeltraud Rohnfeld*
*Translated by Anne Oppenheimer*
ISBN 978 1 84819 078 8
eISBN 978 0 85701 056 8

**Chair Yoga**
Seated Exercises for Health and Wellbeing
*Edeltraud Rohnfeld*
ISBN 978 1 84819 184 6 (DVD)

**Seated Taiji and Qigong**
Guided Therapeutic Exercises to Manage Stress
and Balance Mind, Body and Spirit
*Cynthia W. Quarta*
*Foreword by Michelle Maloney Vallie*
ISBN 978 1 84819 088 7
eISBN 978 0 85701 071 1

**Dance and Movement Sessions for Older People**
A Handbook for Activity Coordinators and Carers
*Delia Silvester*
*With Susan Frampton*
ISBN 978 1 84905 470 6
eISBN 978 0 85700 846 6

**Playfulness and Dementia**
A Practice Guide
*John Killick*
*Foreword by Professor Murna Downs*
ISBN 978 1 84905 223 8
eISBN 978 0 85700 462 8

**Comforting Touch in Dementia and End of Life Care**
Take My Hand
*Barbara Goldschmidt and Niamh van Meines*
*Illustrated by James Goldschmidt*
ISBN 978 1 84819 073 3
eISBN 978 0 85701 048 3

# Qigong

## *for* WELLBEING *in* DEMENTIA *and* AGING

STEPHEN RATH

*with* Marcia Rath

Illustrated by LauRha Frankfort

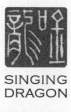

SINGING
DRAGON

LONDON AND PHILADELPHIA

First published in 2016
by Singing Dragon
an imprint of Jessica Kingsley Publishers
73 Collier Street
London N1 9BE, UK
and
400 Market Street, Suite 400
Philadelphia, PA 19106, USA

*www.singingdragon.com*

**Library of Congress Cataloging in Publication Data**
A CIP catalog record for this book is available from the Library of Congress

**British Library Cataloguing in Publication Data**
A CIP catalogue record for this book is available from the British Library

ISBN 978 1 84819 253 9
eISBN 978 0 85701 199 2

Printed and bound in Great Britain

# Contents

# Acknowledgements

We extend our heartfelt gratitude for the many Asian Health practices that shaped this book. After a hip injury, I sought out a gentle exercise and, in 1997, my wife Marcia and I taught ourselves the T'ai Chi Yang Long Form using a video by Terry Dunn. With our interest piqued, we next took classes from Joe Brady of the Tai Chi Project in Denver, and teachers Jason Brown and Master Xilin Zhu. Since 1999, I have continued to study Qigong with Master Zhu and have dedicated over 10,000 hours of practice to the cultivation of vital energy. Through our daily practice, we have experienced the restorative power of Qi; and, as our proficiency grew, we regaled my mother with the forms we were learning. Little did we know that if she had joined along in some movements with us, it might have eased her emerging dementia.

In 2010, a friend taught Marcia two simple Qigong exercises, which immediately healed a health issue. I had been talking about the author of the exercises since meeting him in 2008. And now, Marcia wanted to meet this man. She signed us up for seminars every time he came to Denver. His exercises were so effective that, in 2012, Marcia convinced me to train with him and his coaches, Lynn Thomas, Wade Shigemasa, Pua and Jimmy Kekina, and Mark Siket and others. We became certified to teach many of his exercises. Later, we were fortunate to be invited back to observe and participate in classes taught through his Natural Healing Research Foundation (NHRF), where a cadre of dedicated volunteers have been teaching and educating Hawaiians, especially seniors, in the ways of natural healing since 2006. In the Daoist tradition this humble man simply wants to be known as Grandmaster, and he generously shares his knowledge so that others may benefit from his journey.

The rest of the story unfolds from conversations Marcia and I had with Grandmaster in 2012 about our families' history of dementia. We are enormously indebted to him and to everyone at the NHRF for their generous support, contributions to the exercises and nutrition sections, and for sharing their collective wisdom in the true Aloha spirit; a plenitude of thanks to Pua and Jimmy, who were available day and night to take our phone calls and provide detailed answers to questions about the exercises; the volunteers—Kathie Ong, Pua and Jimmy, Kathleen and JC Coelho, Joan Stone and Gwyneth Ching—who worked tirelessly with us to ensure that the exercise instructions were correct; and, lastly, to all of the other volunteers who work behind the scenes, including a special and deep thanks to Ann Yamamoto, Millannie Akaka, and, of course, Ruby.

To those who gave their time to read and offer valuable feedback to the text through its many revisions, we single out Janet Caldwell, Ann Long, Lynn Thomas, Joan Stone, and Emily Rath for our sincerest thanks. And, Scott and Cindi, our deepest sympathies go out to our innermost circle of family and friends who listened to our many "book" conversations.

We also express deep gratitude to LauRha Frankfort for bringing the text to life with her lively, anatomically correct drawings. Moreover, her inclusion of the ghostly images of the animals in the Five Animal Forms was nothing short of inspired. And, we give Jimmy and Emily a standing ovation for their spirited renditions of the animals illustrated in the Five Animal Forms.

We are grateful to photographers Christine Fagan, Tobias Huber, Jenna Raskin, Tatiana Timmins, and Karen Carver, as well as Cassondra Fischer (graphic artist), who added their talents to the book. We thank Jane Pronovost, Ashley Beck, and LauRha Frankfort for the modeling used in the illustrations.

We give our greatest appreciation for the unwavering support of our publisher, Jessica Kingsley, for her vision and wisdom in seeing the importance of blending two seemingly distant subjects, Qigong and dementia; Rachel Menzies, Commissioning Editor, for shepherding us with kind regard and timely responses from our initial submission to the manuscript's production; and finally, Kate Mason (Production Editor extraordinaire), Sarah Hamlin (Editorial Assistant), and their colleagues, for their very fine work and responsiveness to our many, many revisions in copyediting and design.

With enduring gratitude I thank my T'ai Chi Master and good friend, Xilin Zhu. During the editing process, Zhu played an indispensable role by translating large portions of the book into Chinese in order to bridge the language differences of two cultures. And we offer many thanks to Dr. Shi Cheng, who graciously confirmed our understanding of TCM.

No words can adequately express our humble appreciation for the Grandmaster who so generously gives of himself so others can find wellbeing. Our thanks for all to a truly remarkable man.

Lastly, the greatest contributor to this book is my loving wife and partner in all things—Marcia. Her life and energy animate every page, from her exhaustive research, formatting, and editing to her contributions in Part III. I dedicate this book to her and our mothers, KG and Olive.

# Disclaimer

The exercises and recipes in this book are in no way to be considered as a substitute for consultation with a medical practitioner, and should be used solely at the reader's discretion in conjunction with approved medical treatment. The authors and the publisher are not responsible for any harm or damage to a person, no matter how caused, as a result of following any of the suggestions in this book.

# Qi = Life Force, Energy, Breath
# Gong = Exercise

**Qigong** (pronounced *Chee Kung*) is a modern word for the centuries-old practice of using postures, exercises, breathing, and meditations to improve one's internal energy. The smooth flow of Qi (energy) throughout the meridian channels of the body promotes health and longevity.

The practical exercises, called Gongs, in Part II of this book use movement, sounds, proper alignment, meditation, and abdominal breathing to promote the smooth flow of energy based on relaxation and release. They are intended to ground the energy and bring about a sense of calm.

Many of the Qigong practices described in this book are historically linked to original Chinese Daoist Qigong, dating back to the Jin dynasty (265–420 CE). Daoist Qigong is considered by some to be the basis of Chinese medicine that has been used for thousands of years.

# Preface

One summer night in New England I was practicing T'ai Chi when I received an urgent message to visit my mother, who lived nearby. Arriving at my mother's house, a sensitive woman, Grace, was standing in the driveway. She choked back tears as she described how, on her very first night as a caregiver for an Alzheimer's patient, my mother had inexplicably flown into a rage and kicked her out of the house.

We called her supervisor on my cell phone, who said casually, "Oh, that's no problem. Just go back in the house. She's probably forgotten all about it."

Grace insisted she never wanted to work for my mother again, and she wanted me to drive her home; but, with the combined incentives of the mosquitoes that swarmed around us, and my reassurances, she was persuaded to go back into the house and give Regina's advice a try. When we walked through the door, my mother smiled and betrayed no sign whatsoever of her former rage. Grace worked with love and devotion for my mother for the next five years.

I am genetically and temperamentally linked to my mother, grandmother, and aunt. All of these grand ladies passed away from Alzheimer's disease. For six years I watched my mother, Karen—pianist, environmentalist, world traveler and philanthropist—wither and die. I write knowingly, then, about the stages of cognitive decline. And little did I know at the time that my keen interest in T'ai Chi and the family history of dementia would become inextricably linked.

My wife, Marcia, also knows the stages of dementia. During the period of Grace's employment, Marcia would invite her own mother to join us at our cottage on the Slocum River. Even at age 83, her mother, Olive, would make the four-hour drive from Maine to Massachusetts, skillfully wending her way through Boston's notorious traffic. Once she arrived, she would make a beeline for the back porch, plop down in a rocker with a deep sigh, and count the swans on the far shore. Then she would spend hours in the same chair doing Sudoku, soaking up the sunlight—she had to have her vitamin D—until we would drag her away for dinner. Arguably, this was her favorite spot on the planet. But things changed fast. Three years later we drove her from Maine to our cottage and, as we arrived, she asked with fear and confusion where we were.

In the final stages of dementia, Olive lived in a private home, lovingly cared for by Liz, Chaz, and Max. Forgotten were her productive years as a mother and businesswoman, as well as her life as an artist and folk painting instructor who generously shared her gift. Yet even through her late-stage symptoms of dementia, she would tenderly hold Chaz's hand, and once, even asked him to dance. When she saw our faces coming through the door, her attentiveness and "monkey laugh" of joy were priceless.

If there is anything hopeful to write from our personal story, it is that over the years we have become certified to teach many healing Qigong forms. After participating in a Qigong workshop in Hawaii, we were invited back by the Daoist—who simply wants to be known as "Grandmaster"—to observe his teachers, students, and their family members at his Qi Center in Oahu. We learned about a natural healing program that is ideal for people with memory loss and those at risk of it. Volunteers from his Natural Healing Research Foundation (NHRF) demonstrated programs and shared the invaluable knowledge they impart to people who come from near and far on the island of Oahu. They are remarkable teachers who have worked tirelessly with hundreds of seniors (see page 157). We pay tribute to the success of both the volunteers and the seniors by chronicling some of their stories here. It is no exaggeration to say that their collective efforts are the model from which this book has sprung.

The NHRF has refined and reformatted a series of ancient Chinese exercises to rejuvenate the entire body. Students have reported improvements with cancers, arthritis, strokes, and AIDS, among other health issues, using the exercise and nutrition program. The NHRF more recently recognized that the Qigong practices also proved beneficial for individuals experiencing dementia-related memory loss. For individuals desiring to change their minds, literally, students do hand and feet exercises that bring increased blood and oxygen to areas of their bodies that have grown stagnant and weak. These gentle exercises in the NHRF Senior Wellness Program work because of their simplicity and soft movements.

The book is also designed to help caregivers experiencing stress and burnout. Caregiver burnout can seem as afflictive as dementia, and in fact worry—an emotion commonly experienced by caregivers—has itself been shown to contribute to the development of dementia (see p.53). When the caregiver and person with dementia practice together, the methods in this book can demonstrably provide natural healing for both.

> *It has been so interesting to see the very positive reactions that Marcia has in her Qigong group...how light the mood becomes for each individual resident, as well as collectively in the group...how well the residents participate and respond to the exercises.*
>
> Christine Hendrick, Former Director, Clare Bridge of Highlands Ranch

During the time that Marcia and I spent in Hawaii, we interviewed dozens of people who had a variety of ailments, including seniors experiencing various stages of memory loss. And within two short months of returning home, Marcia began teaching the Exercises for the Aging Brain from the NHRF Program to residents in memory care facilities in Colorado, based upon her experiences and wisdom gained in Hawaii. Many of the seniors who came to class twice a week started to engage actively in the healing sounds, sitting exercises, and hands and feet movements. Moreover, many remembered the exercises from week to week and enjoyed doing them. The residents even invited their caregivers and family members to join in. Marcia exclaimed: "After several weeks a woman, who usually stayed slumped over and unresponsive in her wheelchair, began to rock her feet from side to side one day in an exercise called yin-yang feet—my heart sang for her success."

This book offers exercises from the NHRF's Senior Wellness Program, along with nutritional suggestions and an overview of the research that supports why you or others would use these complementary approaches for wellbeing. The essence of Qigong is to find the quiet within to let our bodies use that quiet to promote wellbeing. Take the first step of doing a few of the exercises for a few days. Know that those steps are continuing a healing art that has been practiced for thousands of years. Feel what happens inside of you and go from there.

Always keep in mind to check with your doctor to see if this program is suitable for you, or someone under your care, before using the natural healing suggestions in this book. If you are sick or weak, you need to see your doctor because this program is not a medical treatment.

# Introduction

*'All things are difficult before they are easy.'*

Chinese Proverb

What is the essence of natural healing? Where can it be found? Perhaps you can find it in the alternative medicine aisle of your local grocer. Or, perhaps it can be found in exercises that have been passed down for thousands of years in China. How much time will it take? And how much will it cost? Will you need special clothes or an exercise machine with a built-in computer and TV screen?

The answer might surprise you: the essence of natural healing lives within you. It is your birthright and path to wellness. The essence is as indispensable to you as your DNA, so that everything else—the foods, herbs, and exercises—are merely the means to unblocking and promoting the natural healing in yourself or the person you are caring for. The essence is known by various names: vital energy, life force, prana, or Qi (pronounced *chee*).

"That may sound all well and good," you say to yourself, "but in practical terms, how will natural healing help my 81-year-old mother who has dementia? How can she do exercises when she can barely stand up and gets feisty at the mere mention of exercise?"

Okay, let's answer those questions by seeing how she would experience natural healing on a daily basis. Can your mother sit? Can she clasp her hands together and rub her palms to generate warmth? Can she stretch her arms up or even just watch as you stretch your arms above your head? Just from watching, she will become engaged in the activity and interact at some level of personal connection. You say she's feisty… Can she pretend to be a tiger and make a GRRRR sound? Can she drink goji berry and walnut oil tea, or eat duck soup? You would be surprised by what natural healing can do for her—and for you.

"But wouldn't it be easier if she just took a pill?" you wonder.

It would indeed be easier for your mother to take a pill, but the results may not be easier to live with. Current medications can provide genuine relief from afflictive emotions and behaviors for some, but only half of the people using prescription medications experience a lessening of symptoms associated with Alzheimer's disease and other forms of dementia (see pages 23–4). Moreover, these medications are not cures and do not affect the outcome of the disease. The treatment modalities have focused on palliating or lessening the symptoms of cognitive decline, including the behaviors associated with it, such as sundown syndrome, agitation, and wandering. But the results are generally modest because the underlying causes have not been addressed. In the following pages, we will explore how Qigong addresses the root causes of memory loss by bolstering the organ energy that supports cognitive functioning. In conjunction with Western medicine, this marriage of approaches may achieve better results to enhance overall health and wellbeing.

One woman who was experiencing acid reflux illustrates how Eastern and Western approaches can be combined. She was prescribed medication by her medical doctor and told she had to take it for he rest of her life; by contrast, her doctor of Traditional Chinese Medicine (TCM) recommended, "Yes, take that medication for a while but also do exercises and take herbs that will support your liver and kidneys. Later, we'll see if you can wean yourself off the prescription medication." Both approaches addressed the need to reduce the acid eating away at her esophagus, but the latter used the body's own healing power to restore health. And indeed, after several months her medication was cut in half, thus lessening the burden on her liver.

The method of natural healing presented here joins together three Eastern practices from the same root, beginning with Qigong (pronounced *chee kung*), a healing practice from China based on a 4,000-year-old natural science. In this book natural healing is the umbrella under which these three approaches to health and wellbeing, including TCM, T'ai Chi, and Qigong, exist. During the senior classes at the NHRF Qi Center, we observed folks who ranged in age from the old to old-old to the oldest doing natural healing exercises with joy and dignity—the energy in the room was electrifying.

# Qigong

Qigong is a healing art that developed over several millennia through observation, study, and proven results. T'ai Chi is a popular form of Qigong and is so effective as a 'supreme ultimate' form of exercise, meditation, and self-healing that it has become the focus of serious study and practice in major universities and hospitals, as reported in the Harvard Medical School Guide to T'ai Chi:

> T'ai Chi is helping to transform Western health care toward integrative medicine. Claims of T'ai Chi's health benefits are increasingly evidenced-based, with more than 700 peer-reviewed, scientific publications in print and more than 180 randomized trials conducted, to date. You might say that T'ai Chi plays an ambassadorial role, helping to integrate Eastern and Western approaches to maximize health. (Wayne and Fuerst 2013, p.282)

Qi is defined as the vital essence or life force that animates all living things and Gong means exercise or work; so Qigong means vital energy work. As early as the Shang Dynasty (1600–1045 BCE), traditional Chinese medical practitioners diagrammed twelve channels in the body, known as meridians, through which vital energy flows to organs and every living cell. Where stagnation or blockages exist in these channels—through injury, trauma, or lack of activity—disease follows. Therefore, Qigong is a practice that moves Qi energy through the meridians to help with health and vitality. These practical exercises commonly use breath, movement, proper alignment, and meditation to improve the flow of Qi. For people concerned with memory loss or those with symptoms of dementia, this book provides gentle and easy exercises and healing foods that support the remaining abilities of people experiencing dementia and advancing age.

---

*With Qigong you feel immediate results, but, Grandmaster never disturbs what your doctors want to do.*

82-year-old Hawaiian

---

If you have not heard of Qigong, you may nevertheless be familiar with acupuncture, which, like Qigong, is taught and practiced as complementary medicine in major medical schools and hospitals throughout the United States and the world, including the Universities of Harvard, Stanford, and Cambridge. Both Qigong and acupuncture stimulate the body's Qi to promote a smooth flow of energy through the body. Though recommended, it is not necessary to attend classes in order to perform Qigong exercises and follow the dietary recommendations. Natural healing exercises are easy to do and can be learned from a book like this: they can be practiced individually, with a loved one, friend, or caregiver; furthermore, the exercises can be practiced at home, in the park, at a community center, or basically anywhere. When people feel the result of Qi flowing in their bodies, they naturally want to do more—in other words, relief brings belief.

## Traditional Chinese Medicine

In order to put into practice the tools of natural healing, it is helpful to understand the simple, yet profound, principles upon which TCM is based. Many people are familiar with the yin–yang symbol and can associate at least one of the opposite—yet complementary—pairs: for example, female and male. They may further know that yin is associated with qualities that are cool, soft, dark, wet, and contracting; while yang is associated with things that are warm, hard, light, dry, and expansive. By simply observing in nature where and how yin and yang exist, the Chinese developed an understanding of the interdependence of these energies and how they continuously transform into each other. This is represented by the tadpole-like shapes of opposite colors in the yin–yang symbol, black and white, which are inextricably linked. But there is also meaning in the smaller circle embedded in each half of the opposite color; it is a reminder that inherent in the qualities of yin and yang there exists an essential part of the other.

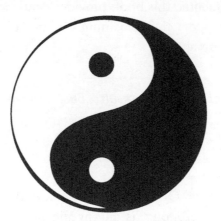

*Figure I.1. The yin–yang symbol*

What many people may not know is that our major organs are comprised of yin–yang pairs and that Qi flows from energy centers (known to the Chinese as the three dantians) through the organs according to a daily cycle. A core tenet of TCM is that these organ pairs depend on a balance of yin and yang energy between them. Therefore, the organs are interdependent and require the support of their opposite in the pair to maintain health: yin organs— liver, heart, spleen, lung, and kidney—are organs that "regulate and store fundamental substances such as Qi, blood, and body fluids"; the paired yang organs—gallbladder, small intestine, stomach, large intestine, and bladder—generally consist of empty cavities and are "responsible for digesting food and transmitting nutrients to the body" (Shen-Nong 2006b). One other meridian pair, the pericardium and triple warmer, function like organs energetically but will not be explored for the purposes of this book. For all of the yin–yang organ pairs, an imbalance of energy in one of the pair of organs invariably leads to an opposite extreme; during illness, for example, an excess of heat during a fever will lead to chills and shivering to cool the body down.

Where there exists a blockage or disruption in the flow of energy, stagnation and illness can occur. A simple analogy illustrates this: if your garden is watered by a sprinkler system that runs according to a daily schedule, but there is a clog or broken sprinkler head in one of the zones along the pipeline, then the plants in that zone will wither and decline. Moreover, if the plant beds are linked together, then a disruption in the flow of water to one zone will ultimately affect another one down the line. In a similar fashion, your organs—the plant beds in this analogy—are energetically linked through channels known as meridians, and a disruption of flow to, say, the kidney, will likewise affect the flow of energy to your heart. The energy of both organs may then decline. This gives a whole new meaning to the popular phrase, "go with the flow."

## Five Element Theory

The Chinese observed the basic elements of nature and developed a philosophy, known as the Five Element Theory, to describe organs and their connection to the basic components of nature. The theory lists the organs in relation to the Five Elements and explains their functional interdependence:

Wood (Liver, gallbladder)

Fire (Heart, small intestine)

Earth (Spleen, stomach)

Metal (Lung, large intestine)

Water (Kidney, bladder)

In the study of TCM, the Five Element Theory describes functional relationships between the elements that are mirrored in the organs of the body. For example, Water is the element in nature that is associated with the Kidney and therefore promotes the Wood of Liver. If there is a deficiency of Water in the Kidney, Wood will not grow properly and the Liver will suffer (see page

69); on the other hand, if there is an excess of Water from the Kidney (high blood pressure), it will douse the Fire of the Heart and harm that organ.

Through empirical observation, then, the ancient Chinese conceptualized the process by which the energy of one organ affects other organs in the body. Additionally, they found that each organ embodies its own unique Qi and is associated in the Five Element Theory with an element of nature, emotion, color, and season—to name a few of the main categories:

TABLE I.1. FIVE ELEMENT THEORY

| ELEMENT | ORGAN | EMOTION | SEASON | COLOR |
| --- | --- | --- | --- | --- |
| **WOOD** | Liver | Anger | Spring | Green |
| **FIRE** | Heart | Joy* | Summer | Red |
| **EARTH** | Spleen | Worry | Late summer | Yellow |
| **METAL** | Lung | Grief | Autumn | White |
| **WATER** | Kidney | Fear | Winter | Dark blue |

*According to TCM, Joy is the emotion of the Heart and is not associated with delight or happiness, as it is commonly understood in the West. Rather, Joy can be either positive or negative and, in excess, creates an imbalance of heart energy.

In TCM joy, for example, can refer to a state of agitation or overexcitement, rather than elation. Related to the heart, this emotion is correlated with heart palpitations. (Pacific College of Oriental Medicine)

In this book, the word Joy will be listed in the charts and text as the Five Element emotion of the Heart, except when Agitation is used to describe an afflictive emotion related to imbalanced heart energy.

In today's world of supercomputers, biochemistry, and synthetic molecules, the Five Element Theory may strike our modern sensibility as rudimentary, even quaint. But the Chinese captured something essential and enduring. The presence of air and water in our daily lives may make them seem unremarkable—but how long can we survive without them? Similarly, Qi may seem mysterious or arcane, but without it we also cannot survive. TCM's grasp of Qi and its relationship to the cosmos helps us understand the relational and dynamic properties of nature, including our own.

Throughout this book, the Five Element Theory describes memory loss from a natural healing perspective and offers suggestions that may help to rejuvenate health and cognitive functioning. In contrast to Western medicine's approach to dementia-related memory loss, natural healing demonstrates that the whole being should be considered. For example, the NHRF observed that people who stoop forward with their necks jutting out may be revealing more about their personal makeup than just poor posture. To a proponent of natural healing, it would further suggest a decline in vital energy and impingement on blood flow and oxygen to the brain from skeletal misalignments. Western medicine might view symptoms like these as unrelated to cognitive decline, whereas natural healing would see them as potential indicators of organ decline that, left untreated, could lead to dementia. Furthermore, natural healing would add a supportive layer of holistic care to the current modality of prescribing drugs for the relief of symptoms; it would also seek to address the root causes of memory loss by correcting skeletal imbalances and improving the organs that affect cognitive functioning.

## About this Book

In the following pages, this book will chronicle individuals who have coped with dementia and other age-related diseases, as well as the natural healing measures they tried. An understanding of natural healing, therefore, will aid anyone interested in developing ways to support the care of those who exhibit symptoms of dementia—or seek to prevent memory loss in themselves.

Chapter 1 provides an overview of how dementia manifests symptoms of decline, not just in the brain, but also in the organ energy that promotes and supports brain functioning. Dementia is described from the perspective of both Western medicine and TCM, with an overview of the functional interdependence of the organs and the manner in which disharmony in one organ can affect the others. Chapter 2 chronicles the stories of seniors with dementia-related indicators, including one remarkable 91-year-old woman whose health, memory and behavior deteriorated after cancer; but with the loving help of her husband, daughter, and other family members, she has experienced the rejuvenating power of natural healing along with allopathic care. Chapter 3 describes the emotional issues that commonly present challenges for individuals, family members, and caregivers. Chapter 4 addresses the special needs of caregivers and provides powerful tools to help them to rejuvenate themselves. The Conclusion draws from elements of the previous chapters and ties them together in the broader context of natural healing.

Part II of this book, "Awaken Natural Healing," introduces the NHRF Senior Wellness Program for the Aging Brain with explanatory text and illustrations, and Part III provides a list of specific foods, recipes, and herbs that may encourage natural healing throughout the body. The intent of these materials is to provide life-affirming assistance to families, medical advisers, and caregivers in their efforts to help loved ones and those who are experiencing memory loss.

In applying the natural healing ideas to help someone with dementia or as preventative care, having the intention to restore whatever vitality is possible, rather than as a method to manage decline, will add positive energy to the effort. For those of us in the Western world, belief in the effectiveness of natural healing may take a leap of faith. But the Chinese have known and practiced mind/body connections for thousands of years in ways that Western science is just beginning to understand, accept, and advocate. Harvard Medical School, for example, has published *The Harvard Medical School Guide to T'ai Chi*, a handbook that offers a twelve-week program on how to live longer and better through the practice of T'ai Chi (an exercise form of Qigong). Therefore, the value of natural healing through Qigong could be summed up in the phrase "changing your mind" and understood as both the need for changing the health of the aging brain, as well as changing attitudes that limit our understanding of the body as its own natural healer.

Natural healing can be used in conjunction with most Western practices, and solutions that afford the most beneficial results—from whatever source— are best. Before you begin this program, your primary care physician or health care provider needs to review the suggestions for exercises and healing foods in this book, to ensure that the suggestions are compatible with the doctor's overall care. In addition to promoting health, the following materials will deepen the bond between the caregiver and the person with dementia. The best benefits accrue when the exercises are practiced as a part of daily living.

---

*I must emphasize that there is no "magic bullet" and one must practice consistently and diligently to gain the full benefits of Qigong...In my case I never want to go back to how I was, so it's easy for me to keep on track...I want to live a long and quality life. It's easy if you keep on doing it.*

82-year-old gentleman

---

# PART I

## A NATURAL HEALING
## Approach to Dementia

# 1

# Western and Traditional Chinese Medicine Perspectives on Dementia

From an early age we learn to name the things of this world. As we develop control over our bodies, feelings intertwine with events and we experience a growing sense of connection. With advancing age, however, this trend may slip into reverse. The fabric of memory can begin to tear when a person feels lost in a familiar location, tells the same story again and again, or forgets important details, places, or events. With further decline a person might forget even the most intimate ties, including lifelong bonds with a spouse, relative, or friend.

According to Traditional Chinese Medicine (TCM), the indicators of decline show up not just in the brain but also in the organ energies from the kidney, spleen, and liver that promote brain functioning. It is no coincidence, then, that memory problems begin in some people who experience nocturnal enuresis (kidney/bladder, liver, spleen—for further explanation, see page 32), digestive problems (liver), or worry and confusion (spleen), to name a few. Changes in mood or behavior, such as anxiety, aggression, and depression, are also significant markers for the onset of dementia.

> A 71-year-old woman suffered many years from anxiety and depression, but after two months of natural healing classes, she reported: *My anxiety reduced to almost a complete sense of wellbeing...and my calmness lasts all day without anti-anxiety and depression medications.*

Prescription medications are commonly used to lessen symptoms associated with dementia and to enhance cognition, but they also carry warnings about their use. As was widely reported in *USA Today* (Marichione 2011) and other media outlets, the current class of medications for the treatment of symptoms (Cholinesterase and Memantine) "works for half who try them and for less than a year on average." Add to that the Food and Drug Administration (FDA) warnings about the side effects for those medications (Doctors Health Press Editorial Board 2005), and one should use appropriate caution when considering whether to use these medications. Natural healing can be used as an effective complement to medications because Qigong may allow the prescriptions to be reduced, or discontinued altogether (Sancier 1999). Moreover, since many medications are processed through the liver, reducing the amount taken may lessen the burden on the liver and its functioning.

When a person with dementia begins to follow a program of natural healing, vital energy can build up day by day and circulate throughout the organs of the body. Common sense dictates that natural healing does not work the same way for all people, or the same way for all stages of memory loss. Rather, natural healing strives to provide complementary care for people who are being treated by Western medicine and, where possible, to rejuvenate the energy of organs that support brain functioning. It is a process that includes the person under care along with loved ones, caregivers, and the community at large—all involved in a widening circle of support.

In the care of most illnesses, including dementia, many TCM experts typically use an approach that effectively combines both Eastern and Western health practices. With certain cancers, the use of radiation and chemotherapy is necessary to destroy cancer cells, even though they wipe out normal cells in the process; this damages organs and sometimes taxes the body beyond what can be sustained. It also confirms the catchphrase that the cure is sometimes worse than the disease. In order to promote the complete health and wellbeing of the individual, natural healing includes techniques that maintain the essential healing qualities of sleep and appetite that are needed during patient care.

> After years of using both approaches to treat patients, I think the answer is this: in traditional Chinese medicine, we consider cancer a local reflection of an overall imbalance in the body. So we fight disease by improving the immune system and increasing energy flow through the meridians. Western medicine, on the other hand, attacks the cancer itself with less regard to other parts of the body…In my experience I have found that a combined approach is preferable.
>
> (Liu with Perry 1997, p.83)

TCM uses the same approach for people with indications of dementia, as well. To those care providers, dementia is not a stand-alone illness in the brain but has its roots in the energy of the organs of the body.

## Kidney

In Traditional Chinese Medicine, the Kidney is considered to be the foundational organ from which our inherited vital essence is stored. It is the root source of our yin and yang Qi and governs physiological functions, such as filtration of the blood, regulation of fluids, reproduction, formation of marrow, health of hair and bones, hearing, and memory. Functionally, the Western understanding of the kidney parallels the Chinese view:

> The kidneys' function are to filter the blood. All the blood in our bodies passes through the kidneys several times a day. The kidneys remove wastes, control the body's fluid balance, and regulate the balance of electrolytes. As the kidneys filter blood, they create urine, which collects in the kidneys' pelvis—funnel-shaped structures that drain down tubes called ureters to the bladder.

(WebMD 2014)

In both TCM and Western medicine, there is a well-known connection between kidney disease and memory problems. Unfiltered toxins in the blood can reach the brain and affect the nervous system. Moreover, the aging process in some people from "old to old-old to oldest" can diminish their kidneys' ability to produce a hormone necessary for the production of red blood cells, which can bring about a corresponding loss of memory and cognition. Natural healing, then, seeks to remedy the energy of the organs that promotes brain functioning and thus reverse the symptoms associated with dementia.

TCM has long understood that the formation of disease happens when the flow of vital energy to the organs is blocked. The same instability in the organs that causes diseases like cancer also affects the functional workings of the brain. Western medicine similarly describes the manner in which dysfunction in the kidneys is believed to play a central role in cognitive decline: red blood cells produced in the bone marrow nourish the brain and other organs with oxygen while carrying away waste in the form of carbon dioxide; however, a decline in a kidney hormone, erythropoietin (EPO), necessary for the production of red blood cells negatively affects the organs, including the brain.

The National Kidney and Urologic Diseases Information Clearinghouse (NKUDIC) illustrates this connection:

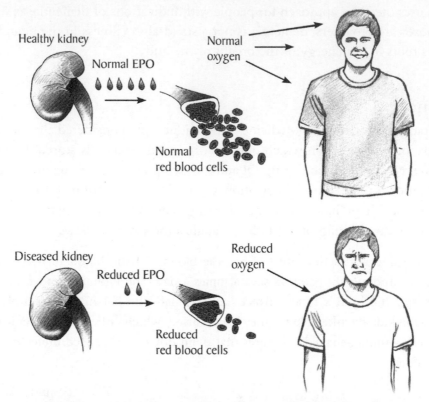

*Figure 1.1. Healthy kidneys produce a hormone called erythropoietin, or EPO, which stimulates the bone marrow to make red blood cells needed to carry oxygen throughout the body. Diseased kidneys don't make enough EPO, and bone marrow then makes fewer blood cells.*

(National Institute of Health 2012, p.1).

In addition to causing anemia, deficiency of red blood cells reduces the amount of oxygen that reaches the brain, so brain cells die, with a corresponding loss of cognition and memory. Drawing a link between diminished oxygen and a gene that triggers a build-up of protein plaques (known as beta-amyloids), a 2006 study (Edelson 2006) published in the National Academy of Sciences advances a likely mechanism in the formation of Alzheimer's disease.

Deprived of oxygen, a cascade of physical symptoms develops concurrently with the loss of brain functioning that includes: cold hands and feet, pain in the knees and lumbar region, weakness, blurred vision, trouble breathing, edema, weak libido, and nocturnal enuresis. Emotional symptoms may appear as well, which include fear, anxiety, paranoia, or panic. Because these symptoms are not generally associated with memory loss, they are often overlooked by Western medicine as early warning signs of dementia.

In 2006, Canadian researchers noted that a specific gene, known as "BACE 1," may be to blame for the lack of oxygen to the brain. It generates a certain protein known as "beta-amyloid," which when found in a higher concentration in the brain can lead to a greater build-up of plaque... According to the study's lead researcher, Weihong Song, "If you have less oxygen, you turn up this gene and obviously generate more beta-amyloid [protein]. If you have a higher level of beta-amyloid protein, you form more plaque. If you have more plaque, then you will have dementia."

(Edelson 2006)

At the NHRF Qi Center in Hawaii, we talked with many seniors who have struggled with kidney issues. Their successful improvement implies that they may have warded off memory difficulties as well. Nancy, a 75-year-old woman, developed kidney problems in her forties but began to recover after she started attending natural healing classes that teach the NHRF's exercises. But she had to stop taking classes when the Senior Center in Honolulu closed due to lack of funding. After three months her daughter became alarmed at the decline in Nancy's health and insisted her mom take the classes in another town. It now takes Nancy a total of 90 minutes to drive up the mountain from Honolulu to the classes in Kaneohe and back. The classes themselves take 90 minutes. But the time issue does not bother Nancy at all because of the results she sees—her health is more important.

*I have been enrolled in the NHRF's Qigong class for about a year now, and it's great. I can sleep through the night now, waking up only once in a while to use the bathroom.*

82-year-old woman

Likewise, Charlie had kidney problems and underwent a transplant in 2002. After surgery he was concerned for a time that his health was not getting better. Like Nancy, he began taking classes at the NHRF Qi Center and made steady improvements. His doctor was impressed with his progress; and his wife, Karen, was so inspired by his improvement that she began teaching at the Center. It is interesting to note that many of the seniors who had health issues themselves now devote their time and energy to helping others learn and practice natural healing.

## Spleen

Another organ dysfunction that may contribute to dementia originates in the spleen. In Western medicine the spleen is identified as the organ that primarily collects platelets and white blood cells while reprocessing old red blood cells. TCM describes the function of the spleen in another way. In TCM theory, the spleen is the main producer of Qi. But when the spleen is out of balance, the smooth flow of Qi is disrupted, resulting in stagnation and an accumulation of phlegm (mucus).

> *My runny nose was a long-term problem, and for years I would wake up daily and my nose would run for one to two hours. The facial exercises eliminated the problem. My nose doesn't run anymore, I've stopped worrying, and I sleep all night.*
>
> 73-year-old woman

Excess phlegm moves to the lungs and is discharged as mucus, or to the kidneys, where it is excreted. If these organs cannot move mucus out of the body, then the excess phlegm becomes adipose tissue or fat. The Chinese call this process "dampness evils." It is described as any outside dampness that penetrates the body, like a fog or cold rain, which collects in the internal organs and disrupts the smooth flow of Qi. Symptoms vary from feeling tightness in the chest, to diarrhea or difficulties with urination. In addition to the physical symptoms, emotions such as worry and confusion can also be signs of possible spleen dysfunction. TCM asserts that inside sources of dampness come from diet and inactivity:

> The spleen is said to be at the root of all phlegm production and is involved in the transportation and transformation of body fluids and foods. If the spleen becomes damaged by eating too many sweet foods and getting too little exercise, it will fail in its duty to move and transform waste fluids and foods. Instead these metabolic wastes will gather, collect and transform into dampness evils. If dampness evils endure over time, they will congeal into phlegm, and become fat tissue.
>
> (Shen-Nong 2006a)

Far from causing just a runny nose or cough, phlegm can set in motion a myriad of diseases related to inflammation and obesity. Western research has recently confirmed that people whose diets are high in trans-fats and hydrogenated oils are more likely to develop Alzheimer's disease. In a French study with over 7,000 adults, it was found that of those with metabolic syndrome—a constellation of symptoms including increased levels of blood pressure, blood sugar, and LDL cholesterol, along with excess abdominal fat—were "20 percent more likely to have cognitive decline on the memory test than those who were free of the syndrome" (Doctors Health Press 2011). But, not surprisingly, Qigong has been shown to reduce at least two of the contributing factors implicated in metabolic syndrome, as confirmed in a study that concluded that Qigong can be effective in regulating blood lipids and reducing blood pressure in hypertensive patients (Myung Suk Lee *et al.* 2004). By definition, if one or more of the factors in the constellation of symptoms comprising metabolic syndrome are allayed, then the patient no longer has the syndrome. Consequently, it is vitally important to reduce the kind of chronic inflammation that originates in the spleen and contributes over time to serious diseases such as dementia.

---

This study investigated the effectiveness of Qigong on blood pressure and several blood lipids, such as high-density lipoprotein (HDL) cholesterol, Apolipoprotein A1 (APO-A1), total cholesterol (TC), and triglycerides (TG) in hypertensive patients. Thirty-six patients were randomly divided into either the Qigong group, or a wait-listed control group. Blood pressures decreased significantly after eight weeks of Qigong. The levels of TC, HDL, and APO-A1 were changed significantly in the Qigong group post-treatment compared with before treatment. In summary, Qigong acts as an antihypertensive and may reduce blood pressure by the modulation of lipid metabolism.

(Marchione 2011)

---

## Liver

Western medicine describes the liver's function primarily as a vital organ in digestion that filters blood, "detoxifies chemicals and metabolizes drugs," and "secretes bile that ends up back in the intestines" (WebMD 2009). But the liver may also play an important role in the formation of early onset Alzheimer's, an inherited form of dementia that is rare and often develops in people before the age of 65. Western research has postulated that the beta-amyloid plaques that clog the brain may actually originate in the liver through the expression of a gene that produces a harmful enzyme:

> 'The product of that gene, called Presenilin2, is part of an enzyme complex involved in the generation of pathogenic beta amyloid,' Sutcliffe explained.

'Unexpectedly, heritable expression of Presenilin2 was found in the liver but not in the brain. Higher expression of Presenilin2 in the liver correlated with greater accumulation of beta amyloid in the brain and development of Alzheimer's-like pathology.'

This finding suggested that significant concentrations of beta amyloid might originate in the liver, circulate in the blood, and enter the brain. If true, blocking production of beta amyloid in the liver should protect the brain.

(Science Daily 2011)

TCM describes a similar model of how dysfunction in the liver may contribute to dementia: if the spleen is the main producer of Qi, the liver is the organ that distributes that energy smoothly throughout the body. Therefore, the liver Qi assists the heart and lungs in the flow of blood to the muscles and tendons. If liver Qi stagnates over time, the proper circulation of blood will be impaired and, together with phlegm from the Spleen, can form plaques that affect the brain. Also, where there is dysfunction in the liver, digestive problems can occur that affect the stomach and spleen:

The liver assists in the smooth flow of the stomach and spleen qi, especially. If the liver qi is not flowing smoothly, bile will not be introduced properly and the liver will attack the stomach and spleen. This can result in nausea, vomiting, belching, reflux, chest and hypochondriac pain, even diarrhea.

(TCM Student 2005)

The function of kidney, spleen, and liver energies has been described, along with the role that energy stagnation may play in the formation of dementia. The NHRF has observed some indicators that may arise from dysfunction and offer suggestions to try:

## NATURAL HEALING POSSIBLE INDICATORS OF DEMENTIA

| Observation | Try something like this |
| --- | --- |
| Cold hands and feet | Hand and feet exercises pages 77–91 |
| Tenderness in web area between the big toe and second toes | Massage the tender point with pencil eraser |
| Thick skin on inner side of big toe | Hold big toe between two fingers and twist it back and forth |

| | |
|---|---|
| Insomnia | Lying down meditation page 64 |
| Dry mouth | Bite teeth and swirl tongue pages 119 & 121 |
| Confusion, agitation, anxiety | Animal Forms & Sounds pages 96–100 |
| Incontinence | 12 Sitting Exercises pages 118–129 |
| Stooped posture/lowered head* | Shoulder rolls on page 135 |

*Especially posture from texting and mobile phone 'apps' and games use

## Interdependence of the Organs

The disruption of Qi from the liver to the spleen illustrates TCM's understanding of the interdependence of the organs and the manner in which dysfunction in the liver contributes to the development of diseases like dementia. Based upon the Five Element Theory, TCM conceptualizes a promotional and restraining cycle of energy that describes how energy flows from one pair of organs to another. If there is a disruption in this cycle, through a blockage or stagnation, another organ is adversely affected and becomes symptomatic. Hence, the liver's contribution to the development of dementia can occur both directly, through impairment of circulation and the formation of beta amyloid plaques, and indirectly by restraining Qi to the spleen.

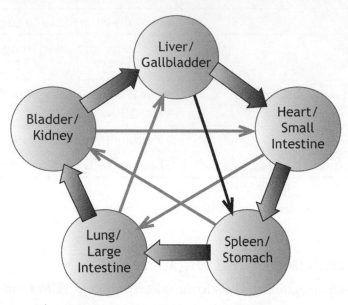

*Figure 1.2. When organs are functioning harmoniously, one pair will promote others in the system, as illustrated by the outer ring of large arrows. But where there exists an excess or deficiency of Qi in one organ, the organ beyond the next one in the series is restrained, as shown by the thin, dark arrows. In this chart, we see how stagnation in the liver restrains the spleen.*

As the spleen becomes restrained, it falters in its ability to process phlegm; this in turn activates the production of fat and inflammation in the body, which, as we have seen, are known factors in the development of dementia. Even a rudimentary grasp of this idea may help in the early detection of dementia, because an understanding of the interdependence of organ energy allows for important signs to be considered in people who develop the disease but do not yet display symptoms of cognitive decline.

Further evidence of the interdependence of the organs can be seen in people who experience nocturnal enuresis. From the perspective of Western medicine, it is due to a weakening of the bladder muscles, which affects bladder control. According to TCM, however, nocturnal enuresis is multi-determined and is a common occurrence for those who experience dementia caused by problems related to organ energy:

1. From the perspective of TCM, spleen energy controls the bladder muscles. When the bladder muscles are weak, this causes conditions such as lack of bladder control and/or inability to empty the bladder completely.

2. Kidney energy—as people age, their kidney energy becomes weaker, which, in turn affects the bladder.

3. Liver energy is most active between 1–3 AM. If the liver energy is imbalanced, one will awaken with the need to urinate.

4. When people's stomachs are empty, or they eat an overly heavy dinner, they may experience sleep problems, since those factors affect their spleen energy. Since they do not sleep well, they also urinate more frequently at night. For males, frequent urination may also indicate problems in prostate.

It can be seen, therefore, that nocturnal enuresis is caused by factors that may indicate not just a weakening of the bladder muscles but also the presence of underlying, and potentially serious, issues in the organs.

In this regard, just by looking at a myriad of physical characteristics—eyes, tongue, skin color, fingernails, movement, to name a few—a doctor of TCM can diagnose internal disorders. Liver problems can be identified by noticing brittle fingernails with little or no moons, skin problems, allergy-like symptoms, sallow eyes, and emotions such as anger and frustration. For TCM, the individual tells the whole story and can be expressed in the adage, "In order to recognize the internal, observe the external – the Zang and the Xiang."

The approach of Western medicine has been to harness state-of-the-art technology to find markers for dementia and answer questions about DNA, biochemistry, and environmental factors. However, Dr. Erica Camargo of Boston Medical Center has uncovered far more simple criteria for determining whether a patient may be at risk for major health problems, including dementia. At the 2012 Annual Meeting of the American Academy of Neurology, she presented her findings that look at hands and feet for answers about how to recognize precursors for dementia and stroke:

These are basic office tests that can provide insight into one's risk of dementia and stroke and can easily be performed by a doctor… The study found that people with a slower walking speed in middle age were one-and-a-half times more likely to develop dementia compared people with faster walking speed. Stronger hand-grip strength was associated with a 42 percent lower risk of stroke or "transient ischemic attack" in people over age 65 compared to those with weaker hand grip strength.

(Marchione 2012)

Dr. Camargo's study affirms the holistic approach favored by proponents of natural healing. In addition to early detection, natural healing seeks to address the root causes of a decline in cognition and offers an approach that restores vital energy to the organs that promote brain functioning. Remarkably, restoring vital energy is easier for seniors to do than one might think. For those who are chair-bound, natural healing offers sitting exercises and healing sounds that demonstrably facilitate blood flow and, in some cases, get these folks back on their feet. Pua, the NHRF Senior Wellness Coordinator at the Qi Center in Hawaii, often receives calls from seniors who tell her, "We can't do exercises standing up." When she tells them that the Center also teaches exercises that can be done while sitting down, they exclaim "Okay!" and sign up for the classes. Soon they find they can do all of the gentle yet invigorating exercises.

As natural healing restores cardiovascular, neural, and energetic pathways, it moves people with failing memories away from a model of care that merely seeks to manage their decline. Instead, the quality of life for some of these folks can be considerably improved, enabling them to feel they have received a second chance to rekindle their sense of wellbeing and the connections that nourish their lives.

# 2

# Examples of the Rejuvenating Power of Natural Healing

The Qi Center in Hawaii is on the second floor of a building with offices that form a square overlooking the plaza below. A woman with a smiling round face and ponytail is skipping backwards on the walkway, beckoning her 91-year-old mother to catch her. The spry mother follows gamely and stretches out her arms to reach her daughter, who is retreating and dancing and gesturing. The courtyard echoes with their laughter.

Maura is the name of the daughter, who is caring for her mother, Beverly. Far from seeing it as a burden, Maura speaks with warmth about the care of both her parents: her mother is a cancer survivor who was diagnosed with Alzheimer's ten years ago, and her father has recovered from a stroke; Maura described that both parents have ongoing consultations with Grandmaster and make regular visits to the NHRF Qi Center.

Maura plays a key part in her parents' rejuvenation. When asked what motivates her to give so much of her time and energy to her parents, she exclaims, "I wanna keep them going!" Her efforts show a remarkable devotion to their wellbeing, although her parents use another term—said with affection, of course—"slave driver!"

Beverly's health issues began to crop up in her late 60s after she retired from managing the family-owned laundromat. Not long after her retirement, she developed throat cancer and had to undergo radiation and chemotherapy. According to Beverly's family, blockages in her neck started a downward spiral in her health that led to cancer and then the onset of dementia: blockages in energy and blood flow between her cervical vertebrae may have contributed to Beverly's cancer; the illness and cancer treatments significantly changed her neck alignment, which caused a further decline in the amount of energy, blood, and oxygen that reached her brain. While taking Chinese herbal supplements, the chemotherapy was successful and Beverly stopped seeing Grandmaster; but later, the family began to notice symptoms of cognitive decline.

"My mother would tell the same story over and over again," Maura reported. "She began to react violently to stuff and accuse Dad of having a lot of girlfriends, even though he was with her 24/7." For Beverly's agitation, her doctor prescribed Risperdal and Namenda. The former was dropped because there were no positive results.

Ironically, although Beverly continued to take the Namenda, the most dramatic improvement occurred after her husband's stroke. When he sought out natural healing at the Qi Center for his care, Beverly went there, too. "My mom's misaligned neck was immediately focused on, because when she first started Qigong, she was hunched over like this," said Maura, leaning forward and stretching her neck out like a turtle. She went on: "It made her off balance and she used Dad as a crutch."

Maura came to understand that her mother's poor posture and loss of balance suggested a classic harbinger of dementia; and, indeed, a quick survey of residents in nursing homes and memory care facilities reveals many people who have forward-leaning postures and necks that jut out. Simply stated, when the vital energy in people declines, they begin to stoop forward. This forward inclination of the head and slouching of the shoulders then impinges on the flow of blood to the aging brain, which increases the symptoms associated with memory loss and behavioral problems. Loss of balance and falling are common problems, and some folks have to be confined to a wheelchair so they don't incur serious injuries.

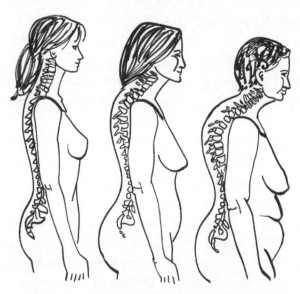

*Figure 2.1. While a slight forward-leaning posture can be a normal part of the aging process, it is comforting to know that many postural problems may be prevented or corrected by consistently practicing natural healing exercises.*

In addition to posture and balance, natural healing looks for points on the body that may show signs that could be developing concurrently with dementia. One such point is the presence of pale and thickening skin on the inside of the big toe (opposite the second toe), which signals a blockage in the neck that might be impeding the flow of energy and blood to the brain. By merely massaging that point, vital energy can begin to bring relief to the afflicted area in the neck. As part of natural healing, then, remedies like these aim to reduce stagnation and disharmonies throughout the system.

The tradition of natural healing has long understood what current research is just beginning to accept: exercises that improve posture and balance also affect positive changes in the mind, body, and emotions. Studies have shown that seniors who are no longer afraid of falling get a tremendous boost to their confidence and self-esteem, not to mention the benefit of increased blood flow and oxygen to the brain.

> *I can now move my body more fluidly...my posture also improved. I have gained a more positive outlook on life and am much more happy, relaxed, and poised.*
>
> 72-year-old

Citing a 2005 University of Chicago study, a report from the World Tai Chi and Qigong Day describes how an "enriched environment" that "includes both learning and physical activity increases the output of genes involved in maintaining the health of neurons, constructing synaptic connections, and building arterial highways to supply more blood to the brain." The report concludes that T'ai Chi (a form of Qigong) may be the ideal exercise for changing the molecular structure of the brain and promoting regeneration:

> T'ai Chi's complex motions which engage left and right brain, mind and body, upper body and lower body, and left body right body motions that require mental awareness to perform in sequence, may make T'ai Chi the most profound exercise to achieve the above results.
>
> (World Tai Chi and Qigong Day, 2005)

Further support comes from the Harvard Women's Health Watch (2009), which describes the health benefits of T'ai Chi as "*medication* in motion."

For her care, Beverly followed the suggestion to join the NHRF Senior Wellness Program, which is described in Part II of this book, and includes: Hand and Feet Exercises, Five Animal Forms, Facial Completion Exercises, and

Twelve Sitting Exercises. Maura credits these exercises for greatly reducing her mother's agitation and memory loss, while increasing the range of motion in her neck. Maura was happy when the NHRF introduced a set of Hand Exercises that also enhance memory by stimulating the liver, kidneys, and neural pathways to the brain. The mechanism of how this works can be summed up in an apt phrase: "Hands Light up the Brain."

However, behind this deceptively simple explanation lies a solid foundation of scientific research that validates the effectiveness of using hand exercises to enhance brain functioning:

> A map of the brain shows that the nerve endings on your fingertips correspond to more areas of the brain than any other body area, except perhaps the tongue and lips. Therefore, finger exercises and movements can be useful in stimulating the neurons in the brain. The National Institute of Mental Health conducted experiments that showed finger exercises enlarged the capacity of the participants' brains, increased connections between neurons, forged new neural pathways, and increased circulation to the brain areas. The researchers concluded that finger exercises contributed significantly to brain plasticity, the ability of the brain to renew itself. Increased circulation means more oxygen and nutrients for the brain cells and decreased waste products that clog up the brain.
>
> (Brain Injury Research Institute 2007)

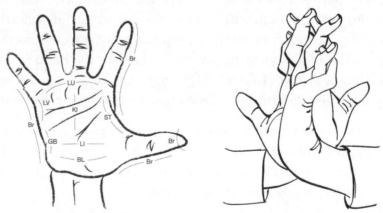

*Figure 2.2 The hand is dotted with reflexology points. Massaging these point areas on the hands by doing hand exercises stimulates a good flow of energy, blood, and oxygen to promote the energy of each organ. 1. LI – Liver; 2. GB – Gallbladder; 3. Heart (located on the left palm in the same area as the Liver); 4. ST – Stomach; 5. LU – Lung; 6. LI - Large Intestine; 7. KI – Kidney; 8. BL – Bladder; and 9. Br – Brain. (Anatomical Chart Co. 1974)*

According to Western medicine, one quarter of the sensory and motor cortex controls the hands. Many brain problems (Parkinson's, dementia, and stroke) show hand symptoms, so some brain functioning may be improved by restoring the natural curvature of the arch of the hand through exercises. The program in Part II of this book includes hand stretches and movements that use "pressure and leverage" to reestablish the hands' natural curvature, strength and flexibility. The Brain Injury Research Institute (2009) encourages people of all ages to move their fingers to improve their brains.

The Western mind has grown accustomed to, and hence is reassured by technologies like magnetic resonance imaging (MRIs) and genetic tests that reveal the essential building blocks of a person's body. In contrast, one advantage of natural healing is that the indicators for problems in the brain are not only observable to the naked eye but can be improved through exercises that promote natural healing. For Maura the results are tangible, because she has seen a noticeable improvement in her mother's abilities compared to friends in their community who do not engage in natural healing:

> The main thing is that when you tell her something, she doesn't forget it right away. Like when you give her instructions. Sometimes, when you're talking with people with Alzheimer's, you tell them something and they forget what you just said. They turn to you every five seconds and ask you the same question.

Equally impressive for Maura is how well her mother is doing with the exercises:

> The best part is that she knows how to do the exercises. She can follow along with what they're doing, and she's already catching on to the new hand exercises that they do in the morning. Now she can do the Rooster's Comb—when she started she couldn't even link her fingers together.

The significance of this development is that Beverly previously could not link her fingers. But with repeated efforts, she has succeeded and now benefits from the resulting changes in her hands. Along with the hand exercises, she does the program's healing sounds, as well as dietary recommendations to support her organ energy. All of these things have calmed Beverly down, improved her ability to remember instructions and exercises and, most importantly, enhanced her quality of life. Given that people with dementia usually develop incontinence, it may be a measure of the natural healing's preventative care that Beverly is once again able to use the bathroom by herself.

Perhaps there is no more dramatic example of the rejuvenating power of Qigong in the recovery of memory than in the case of an 80-year-old man, we'll call Arthur, who experienced repeated mini-strokes. He was frequently disoriented and would "just zone out and forget where he was." Initially, he used acupuncture and herbs, but those did not give him much relief. After two months his acupuncturist taught him a hand exercise known as Rooster's Comb (p.84–85). Arthur practiced this exercise, which simply required that he slide one hand around the other until the backs of the hands were touching with the fingers pointing toward the ceiling; then he linked all the fingers— from the pinky fingers to the index—and extended his hands and arms as high above his head as he could, breathing as instructed by his coach.

Arthur's acupuncture sessions were quickly reduced from three times a week to once a week and, after only six months, the Rooster's Comb seemed to have deepened the effectiveness of the acupuncture and herbs to the point that he no longer needed them. He continued to practice the Rooster's Comb at home. The addition of the Rooster's Comb appears to confirm the simple yet profound adage, "Hands light up the brain."

These same benefits from Qigong accrue to more than just the ailing brains of those with dementia. Several of the seniors found their way to the Qi Center after they had suffered strokes and their aftercare medical benefits had run out. One story brings to mind an adage of Master Kwan of Canton, China: "The trip to my home is proof that a person truly wants to be healed. The climb up the mountain is a great motivator" (Liu with Perry, p. 20).

Metaphorically speaking, one man exemplifies that adage. David 'climbs the mountain' every week, traveling great distances to get to the Qi Center. David is a gentle 75-year-old man who had a debilitating stroke, crippling the entire right side of his body. His daughter, Carol, left her job on the mainland and rushed to his side in Hawaii, convinced he would not live long. Initially, David was wheelchair bound, with his insurance coverage for physical therapy running out, when a friend suggested he visit the NHRF office for a consultation. That began David's journey up the mountain.

One year after his stroke, David confessed during an interview with us that he had previously hoped for a pill that would take care of his problems. Instead, David found that the non-strenuous exercises brought about amazing results. Within 90 days he advanced from a wheelchair to a walker to a cane; and within six months he was walking without a cane. Currently, the only blood-thinning medication he takes is Chinese tea.

Now David is on the top of the mountain. When he spoke to us, there were no visible signs of stroke whatsoever—no contorted mouth, frozen facial features, or awkward movements—nothing. Instead, his eyes sparkled and he smiled often. During the healing sounds portion of class, his gentle voice could be heard roaring out the sounds of a bear, releasing any worries that he might ever be crippled by a stroke again.

The story of Beverly's husband, Emmet, parallels David's in several regards: after his stroke in 2003, he was confined to the house, stuck in a wheelchair with his insurance benefits running out. This was challenging for a man who had served this country honorably during World War II (naval reservist in the 442nd Oriental) and had opened the first market in Honolulu after the war. Emmet was used to being self-sufficient.

Over lunch at a favorite Chinese restaurant near the Qi Center, Emmet was asked how Qigong exercises have helped him the most. He lowered his head and said softly, "I no longer wet the bed." It was not easy for him to talk about. Like David, he shows no signs of ever having suffered a stroke. In the restaurant I strained to hear this quiet and earnest man talk about what was currently on his mind. No longer did he focus exclusively on his health issues but, instead, mourned the loss of buddies who had died during and since the war.

Beverly and Emmet are leading full and healthy lives. Emmet is the eldest member in his Lions club and has returned in his ninth decade to teaching ballroom dancing. Beverly sometimes walks to church and loves to play golf with her husband. They play on a hilly course, and Beverly is not satisfied until she has successfully completed her nine holes game. Gone are the days when she didn't have enough strength or balance to stand upright and had to use Emmet as a crutch. "She doesn't need Dad anymore," Maura says with a peal of laughter—"she just takes off!"

---

These stories are far from unique. The following studies by Dr. Kenneth Sancier Ph.D. (1996) in *Anti-Aging Benefits of Qigong*, cite the effects of Qigong on patients with dementia.

**Reversing symptoms of senility.** To study the mechanism of keeping fit by qigong, a controlled study was made of 100 subjects classified either as presenile or with senile impaired cerebral function. The subjects were divided into two groups of 50 people each with a mean age of 63 years and with a similar distribution of age and sex. The qigong group practiced a combination of static and moving qigong. The control group exercised by walking, walking fast, or running slow... Criteria for judging outcome were based on measuring clinical signs and symptoms including cerebral function, sexual function, serum lipid levels, and function of endocrine glands.

After six months, 8 of the 14 main clinical signs and symptoms in the qigong group were improved above 80 percent, whereas none of the symptoms in the control group were improved above 45 percent. These results suggest that qigong can reverse some symptoms of aging and senility. In this regard, qigong exercise is superior to walking or running exercises.

**Enhanced activity of an anti-aging enzyme.** Superoxide dismutase (SOD) is produced naturally by the body but its activity declines with age. SOD is often called an anti-aging enzyme because it is believed to destroy free radicals that may cause aging. The effects of qigong exercise to treat disorders of retired workers were studied by Xu Hefen and coworkers and included determinations of plasma SOD. For their study, 200 retired workers, 100 males and 100 females, ranging in age from 52 to 76 were divided into 2 groups: the qigong exercise group and the control group, and each group consisted of 50 males and 50 females...

The result showed that the mean level of SOD was increased by qigong exercise. For example, the SOD level was larger in the qigong group (about 2700 $\mu$/g Hb) than in the control group (1700 $\mu$/g Hb), and this difference was significant ($p<0.001$). This study shows that qigong exercise can stimulate physical metabolism, promote the circulation of meridians and regulate the flowing of Qi and blood, thus preventing and treating disorders of aging and promoting longevity.

**Blood flow to the brain.** Qigong exercise has been shown by rheoencephalography to increase blood flow to the brain. For 158 subjects with cerebral arteriosclerosis who practiced qigong for 1 to 6 months, improvements were noted in symptoms such as memory, dizziness, insomnia, tinnitus, numbness of limbs, and vertigo headache. During these studies, a decrease in plasma cholesterol was also noted. These results may offer hope to people with cerebral arteriosclerosis.

People with Alzheimer's often suffer from other ailments. For those interested in natural healing, Dr. Sancier's research is extensive and worth perusing because it validates the benefits of Qigong on important health issues, such as cardiovascular fitness, hypertension, blood flow, cancer, dementia, and general functions of the body.

# 3

# Natural Healing for Emotional Wellbeing

As we have seen, the early stages of dementia can go undiagnosed and are not readily distinguishable from other age-related changes in memory and behavior. It is not until these changes depart from a person's usual patterns—typically during the middle stages—that family members and friends begin to take notice. According to Maura, her mother's behavioral changes started after her cancer:

> She used to fight me a lot after her cancer. What I noticed is that when she got into a fighting mood, if I just went someplace else and came back a little later and changed the subject, she would have forgotten about being feisty and being in that mood. But if I pursued the fight, then she would remember it. I mean, other things would just come and go, but that she would remember.

Maura's reaction to her mother being "feisty" is a good model for others to use in diffusing a difficult situation. Rather than engaging in a conflict, it is sometimes best to withdraw, let the other person "forget about it," and then return a little while later. Beverly's behavior also provides signposts for what may be going on inside of her. As the adage reminds, "In order to recognize the internal, observe the external." This is as true for the afflictive emotions and behaviors of people with ongoing memory loss as it is for their physical symptoms, such as urinary tract infections or aches and pains.

Just as TCM affirms the relationship between organ dysfunction and dementia, it identifies a psychology of emotions based upon the time-tested Five Element Theory and its matching organs. TCM tells us that each organ embodies its own unique Qi and its own unique emotion. If there is an imbalance of energy in one or more of the organs—through genetics, environment, disease, lifestyle, or trauma—there will also be a problem with the corresponding emotion. Thus, alcoholics who destroy their livers are commonly known to be angry; but a vicious cycle ensues because excessive anger further damages the liver. From the perspective of natural healing, releasing afflictive emotions from the organs not only maintains good mental health but may also help to diminish the formation of diseases like dementia (PCOM 2014).

### TABLE 3.1. ORGANS AND THEIR ASSOCIATED EMOTIONS

| | |
|---|---|
| **ANGER** | Over time anger diminishes liver functioning and, conversely, a dysfunctional liver increases anger. If the liver is unable to distribute Qi smoothly throughout the body, disharmony between liver and spleen energy can cause depression. |
| **JOY** (see page 18) | Excessive joy creates agitation. Coupled with kidney problems, disharmony between kidney and heart energy can lead to anxiety, panic attacks, and heart problems. |
| **WORRY** | Worry causes disruption in the functioning of spleen and stomach energy. Likewise, a stomach or spleen disorder can cause worry. |
| **GRIEF** | Constant crying can affect the energy of the lungs, which interrupts the flow of body fluids. |
| **FEAR** | Fear is the emotion associated with the kidney. Energetically, the kidneys are considered to be the bedrock of the body, so strengthening kidney energy promotes support throughout the entire organ system. |

Seemingly aggressive behaviors such as yelling, breaking things, or hitting may be an act of communication for someone who cannot find words or other ways to express bottled-up emotions or internal pain. In addition to a decline in liver functioning, aggression can be exacerbated by a sense of loss of control or physical discomfort. For Beverly, acting "feisty" may have come from her inability to shower or brush her teeth without Maura's help. Before the onset of Alzheimer's, Beverly was quite independent; and now, natural healing has returned a measure of that independence to her life. She is able to manage everyday tasks more easily now, and she even ties her own shoes after class and buttons her clothes.

Also, some of the routines and activities that were once familiar for Beverly may have become confusing and insurmountable. These losses pose even more of a challenge for people when their cognitive decline affects their ability to communicate verbally. For the caregiver, then, recognizing nonverbal cues and body language is an important tool in interpreting a person's needs.

My mother-in-law, Olive, would point her finger at something or tap objects to communicate. She worked with her hands throughout her life—

knitting, sewing, typing and painting—so she was comfortable with the exercises and hand massages that Marcia started to do with her. We believe this improved Olive's pathways to communicate, as well as her hand strength. It was also a constant reminder that even though she had trouble talking, she was still very much cognizant of her inner and outer world. Her ability to utter complete sentences returned sometimes, while at other times she spoke incoherently. At that point Marcia and I joined in a rambling discourse with her; and even if it seemed nonsensical to others, Olive-us (pun intended) enjoyed the conversation and fun time.

The onset of dementia in some people's lives can be deceptive and crushing. For one couple, Ron and Dora, the symptoms appeared in Dora so fast and at such a young age that even her doctors were at a loss to make an accurate diagnosis. Dora was in her late forties when the disease started, but she was not diagnosed until her mid-fifties. As an educational specialist and writer, she possessed a sharp mind. Also, she and her husband led a very active lifestyle—being avid skiers and bicyclists—so a diagnosis of Attention Deficit Disorder (ADD) seemed to fit her age and general profile. For her symptoms she was prescribed Adderall, which appeared to help initially. But her symptoms were episodic and worsened during times of stress, such as when her mother died. When the medication was discontinued, her symptoms remained the same, and then other diagnoses had to be considered to account for her mood swings: was she bipolar or having petit mal seizures?

Inexplicably, she started to lose words and forget how to complete simple tasks. In one telling incident, Ron asked Dora to look up directions on her cell phone while he was driving. When Dora was unable to figure out how to use the phone, Ron became upset. It was then that he began to realize that something very serious was happening to her. As he calmed down, Dora quietly confided to him that she was no longer able to add or multiply.

An autopsy on Dora's 86-year-old mother revealed that she had died from arterial stenosis with Alzheimer's. But what would that have to do with a fit, middle-aged woman with a keen mind? Comprehensive tests were ordered for Dora, including MRI, CAT scan, blood work, spinal tap, and neurological testing. The spinal tap revealed that she was developing Alzheimer's disease.

Ron began taking Dora to the day program at the Memory Care Center. By the age of 60 she needed to be guided through the door and helped into the main hall, where the other residents gathered for their Qigong class. Dora shuffled her feet and walked with a mildly rounded posture, as many with dementia do. Once seated, she would wear a look that seemed to alternate between confusion and fear, and even in the warm room her hands remained cold. Being uncommunicative in other ways, she would sometimes weep uncontrollably. What was Ron thinking during such moments? They had been sweethearts since college. How long ago was it—five, seven years?—they were careening down a ski slope, racing, laughing, and enjoying the moment. What...happened?

---

Researchers at the Washington School of Medicine in St. Louis now believe they have a way to detect whether someone is vulnerable to an inherited form of Alzheimer's, by testing the spinal fluid of people whose parents developed early onset of the disease.

The researchers are following members of families who have mutations in one of three genes:

- amyloid precursor protein
- presenilin 1
- presenilin 2.

People with these mutations will develop Alzheimer's early, between their thirties and fifties, previous research has shown.

The researchers have found a way to predict the age of disease onset among study participants by referencing their parents. For instance, if a parent developed dementia at the age of 50 years, a child who inherited the mutation would be expected to develop dementia at roughly the same age. As a result, scientists have been able to track disease progression, including the many years during which Alzheimer's is active in people's brains but symptoms are not yet visible (Doctors Health Press 2011a).

---

When Dora began the Exercises for the Aging Brain classes at the Memory Care Center, a look of resolve would sometimes flicker across her face. She tried to keep up with the class during the hand exercises, but the class had usually moved on to the next series. At times her hands would grow warm, and to the casual observer it seemed as if she had brief moments of transcendence, when her spirit would break out of its prison house. She sometimes expressed herself through smiles, movement, and hugging; and although Ron wondered if this was a "halo effect," he spoke about how she had begun to participate more and would stand up and roar like a bear during the Five Animal Forms.

With cherishing concern and determination, Ron tried many things that seemed to hold the promise of hope. He even fed Dora the latest miracle food, coconut oil—to no effect. Even with the disappointments, however, he was eager to have Dora do more Qigong exercises because, above all, he saw a quiet dignity returning to her life. He also started to come to class in order to learn and practice the Hands and Feet Exercises with Dora. He particularly liked the animal sounds and was hopeful that the healing sounds might relieve some of the crying that choked Dora's lungs with grief.

Sadly, Dora passed away in her sixty-second year after a sharp decline. The Memory Care Administrator said that early onset Alzheimer's can be very aggressive and that residents often advance through the stages quickly. Although Qigong did not seem to alter the course of Dora's illness, Ron expressed gratitude that it returned some measure of dignity to her life.

Even in people older than Dora, the onset of Alzheimer's can be just as deceptive. One such age-older woman, Ethleen, began to mask signs of cognitive decline before she or others recognized what was going on. Until her mid-eighties she lived alone, drove a car, paid her bills and otherwise managed her life as an independent person. To her family, the forgetfulness and hearing loss that crept in seemed to be mild or age-related. But from TCM's perspective, an impairment of auditory perception is yet another indicator of decline in kidney functioning. Behaviors like hoarding started little by little; her wandering around the house at night seemed to come from loneliness, and her agitation at dinner could be excused as a mood or phase. But these behaviors signaled a state of confusion and anxiety that, sadly, took on added weight in hindsight. Ethleen's daughter, Lois, related how distraught she was that she didn't notice sooner how much her mother's abilities had declined:

> My mother wasn't calling any longer, and I just assumed she was busy or annoyed with me. I never even thought she might have forgotten my number. When I called her, I didn't notice that I was the one bringing up most of the topics. She was good at saying, "Oh yes," and "I can believe that." When she did talk about her goings on, she was full of agitation: "Can you believe those trucks keep coming around the corner and waking me up at night!" She even went to City Hall and told them a thing or two about the trucks.

Lois talked about Ethleen's increasingly eccentric behaviors and how easy they were to dismiss as quirky. Ethleen would get very upset if Lois tried to help with anything, so it seemed prudent for Lois simply to agree and let her mother be. After all, Ethleen had managed her house in her own way for 50 years and Lois felt like a meddler when she suggested a change. Lois compared recognizing signs of mental decline to watching children grow: "They become a foot taller without you ever seeing the inches." Lois finished with emphasis, "And you might not notice all the things about your mother's decline until she comes to live with you and you discover she's been fashioning plastic bags to hide her wetting!"

By the time Ethleen came to live with Lois, Ethleen was in a state of confusion and anxiety. The moment Ethleen walked through the door, she turned on Lois's husband, Luke, and said, shaking her finger, "Are you tricking me? This is just like my daughter's house. She has this same table!"

Luke picked up the story:

> How we convinced Ethleen to go bed that night, I can't remember. By morning she was her old self, enjoying breakfast and teasing the cat. But by late afternoon she'd start with any number of accusations. One evening I came home as Ethleen was slapping her checkbook across her hand and saying to Lois, "You've written in my checkbook! What do you think you're doing? That's not your money. You leave mine alone!"

What Ethleen didn't remember was that she had turned that responsibility over to Lois well before moving in with them.

Another concern was that Ethleen got up at night and just wandered around and around the house for hours, turning the lights on and off. Luke continued his story:

> Sometimes it was creepy to get woken up in the middle of the night like that. I'd try to communicate with her, but she just kept walking her rounds, as if I wasn't there, like she was on remote control.

This reflects a state of anxiety that is typically seen in the middle stages of dementia, and it is reported, "Two characteristic precursors to wandering are restlessness and disorientation" (Smith, Russell and White 2013). Another form of anxiety is manifested in "sundown syndrome," a mood disorder in which people become quite agitated in the late afternoon or into the evening.

Western medicine does not yet understand the mechanism of sundown syndrome, but offers this advice: close the curtains or shades before dusk in order to make a person with dementia less aware of the coming nightfall. In most cases that doesn't seem to help, to which natural healing offers another perspective. As we have seen, Chinese medicine has long believed that organs are repositories of human emotions, with the kidneys holding fear and panic. Since the time of day when vital energy nourishes the kidneys is strongest from five o'clock in the afternoon until seven in the evening—the hours when sundowning and anxiety are at their peak—TCM suggests treating blocked or deficient kidney energy.

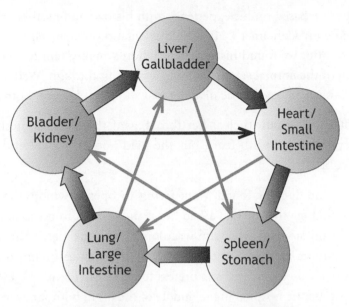

*Figure 3.1. In this chart the thin, dark arrow indicates that the kidney restrains the heart. One example of how emotions in one organ can affect emotions in another is during sundown syndrome, in which fear produced in the kidney at dusk can also affect the emotions of the heart and cause agitation.*

Another woman, Ruth, who was renowned for her level-headedness and wisdom, illustrates some of the misunderstandings that can befall a person with dementia. The needs of this woman became so great after she suffered a silent heart attack that her daughter and son-in-law knew it was no longer safe to have Ruth live in their two-story home, where she had to climb stairs. She had lost her ability to initiate activities and, when alone in a room, she didn't know where she was or what to do. Her agitation around the time of sundown was particularly acute. Lynn and Patrick began looking for a Senior Care facility, and it seemed logical to think that a small private setting with only a half-dozen residents would have the familiarity of home. After all, there was even a pet dog in the residence. What wasn't known at the time was the extent of Ruth's need to wander, and she quickly showed signs of being pent up in the small setting. She grew more agitated, which was her nonverbal way of communicating that something was wrong with her environment. Perhaps Lynn and Patrick should have taken it as a clue when the dog ran away. Lynn bit her lip as she started to explain what her mother had endured:

> The director of the house would call day after day to say Mom was getting into things and batting at people. I didn't know what to do. He said she needed anti-psychotic medications, but when Mom took them she got worse. We had picked that facility in the first place because the director claimed to

have expertise based on his experience with his dad and mother-in-law, both struggling with Alzheimer's. His whole orientation was management through medication. But we found his experience didn't qualify him to know how to handle all of the normal stages my mom was going through. Well, I'll tell you, Alzheimer's isn't a psychiatric disorder and shouldn't be treated that way.

At this point Lynn began to clear her throat, as if there was something stuck there. Her eyes flooded with tears, but she held her gaze level and her voice firm as she continued:

One night the director found Mom trying to open a window in an empty room. He told me that he had asked her if she wanted to go somewhere. She said "yes" and stopped what she was doing. He took her in his car to the emergency room and left her there without so much as giving our name as next of kin. He used her "yes" as a pretext to get her to leave. The ER then sent her to a psychiatric hospital in the middle of the night without even calling us. My mother was left all alone in the ambulance. He didn't go with her. I didn't know until I called him in the morning. I cry when I think how terrified she must have been. And he sent her *alone* to the scariest place I have ever been. I mean scariest. Dark, dingy, smelling of urine. People moaning, crying, scratching at the door. My mother was struggling to get out of a restraining chair. At first Patrick tried to calm her down and divert her attention. He loves her. But she kept trying and trying to break free. After a while he got so depressed and angry he didn't try to stop her anymore. He was trying to will her on. And, you know what, she broke free! My husband cried. He still does.

That same day the chief-of-staff of the psychiatric hospital released Ruth, telling Lynn it "was totally unwarranted" for her mother to have been admitted there. While the disease can create hallucinations and delusions in people who were previously psychologically healthy, the doctor informed Lynn that, in the majority of cases, people with Alzheimer's do not generally need to be admitted to a psychiatric unit unless there was a history of psychosis prior to the onset of the disease. He was angry, and a complaint was lodged with the state against the private care facility. He said he gets tired of seeing Alzheimer's patients being "dumped."

No word yet on the dog.

Once Ruth's need for wandering was met in a senior living home with a staff well trained in behavioral interventions for people with memory loss, she went about her life with much more independence. With Ruth's stress relieved,

Lynn and Patrick could concentrate on restoring the quality of their lives rather than living with the anxiety of facility-induced behaviors.

One important behavioral intervention involved movement, and Ruth's new senior living home had just started a new Qigong class. Patrick was effusive in his praise:

> I'll tell you, if a care place is experienced enough to know people can be helped by doing Qigong, then they are experienced enough for you to consider it as a place for your mother to live. I tried the meditation and talked Lynn into trying. It has done us all a world of good in the calming-down department.

Indeed, research on neuroplasticity of the brain as reported in the *Harvard Medical School Guide to T'ai Chi* (Wayne and Fuerst 2013) has shown that Qigong and T'ai Chi are effective alternative therapies for calming down seniors who are depressed or agitated. Researchers now acknowledge that human brains have the ability to rewire neural connections to enhance health, calmness, and overall wellbeing.

---

Stress, especially chronic stress, can lead to heightened arousal that triggers stress hormones, such as cortisol, that are known to impact brain function. In addition, stress can alter other types of neurotransmitters in the brain, such as serotonin and dopamine, which, along with stress hormones, are linked to depression and other psychological disorders. Multiple active ingredients of T'ai Chi are designed to reduce stress and, therefore, may help you manage stress and mood disorders. The slow, deep breathing associated with T'ai Chi, for example, has been associated with reductions in anxiety and stress hormones.

(Wayne and Fuerst 2013, p.210)

---

The wish of some seniors to "go home" (even if they are home) is another form of confusion and anxiety that occurs in people who do not recognize their surroundings. A compassionate man, Henry, tells the story of his mother, Jane:

> I was visiting Mother at the home she had lived in for ten years. Her caregivers had warned me that she was getting restless, so I was already primed for her to stage a palace coup, break out, and leave the caregivers in the dust. Sure enough, no sooner had I walked through the door than she demanded, "I want to go home!" Since Mother had lived in quite a few different homes throughout her life, I asked, "Which home do you mean?" I was really curious because I wondered if she was longing for her childhood home or some place she remembered fondly. But she replied, "I don't know," and became more

upset. Then it occurred to me to say, "Mother, this *is* your other home. We'll go to the one you want tomorrow." This seemed to calm her down, but I had to wrestle with the fact that I'd told a lie.

Indeed, Henry's discomfort is not unusual. Those who have been conditioned to be honest since childhood may find it difficult to tell "a lie," especially to a parent. People with dementia are sometimes incapable of understanding the literal truth. For example, Jane believed without a shadow of a doubt that there was a place—no doubt ideal in her mind—that was her *real* home. That was her reality. Experts recommend that you enter the world of those who have lost the ability to reason or make sense of their surroundings; it will help you respond more effectively to their needs.

Unfortunately, Jane was not given the opportunity to combine natural healing with her many medications to see what improvements might have occurred in her health and emotions. Although she received excellent palliative care, this once strong woman progressed quickly through the stages of Alzheimer's, finally withdrawing from life completely.

# 4

# Rejuvenation for the Caregiver

Caregiver burnout is very real and has to be factored into the cost, in every sense of the word, of caring for those with dementia. Caregivers sometimes experience difficult emotions, but they may be unwilling to acknowledge or deal with them. The problem is compounded when caregivers hope that the people under their care can be treated through pharmaceutical interventions, only to discover that the symptoms and afflictive emotions continue or get worse. Over time, the day-to-day grind of caregiving, with all of its worries and frustrations, can damage the health and wellbeing of the caregiver.

Indeed, recent research at the Rush Alzheimer's Disease Center at Chicago's Rush University indicates that worry itself can contribute to Alzheimer's:

> People who are prone to psychological distress—negative emotions like worry and anxiety—are more likely to develop memory problems than those who adopt a more carefree existence, according to two studies on aging that together included over 1200 people.
>
> In fact, study participants who experienced negative emotions most often were more likely to develop mild cognitive impairment than those who experienced the least negativity.
>
> (Health Realizations 2013)

Just as we have seen the functional interdependence of organs in the human body, likewise, there is a functional interdependence between a caregiver and a person experiencing debilitating memory loss. Obviously, the person under care depends upon the caregiver for life, sustenance, and wellbeing. But the reverse is also true.

Whether the caregiver is a paid professional, a family member, or friend, the responsibilities of caring can equate to a rewarding but, at times, burdensome experience; in a sense, then, the caregiver depends upon the cooperation of the person being cared for to ensure the smooth running of the work. When that doesn't happen, caregiver emotions may become excessive and create energy imbalances that can turn a normal emotion into an afflictive emotion: anger can escalate to rage; joy can disintegrate into agitation; worry can increase to anxiety; grief can deepen into anguish; fear can intensify into panic.

---

## WHEN NORMAL EMOTIONS BECOME AFFLICTIVE

Afflictive emotions come from excessive or deficient organ energy.

**ANGER:** Angry feelings can arise when the person you're supporting thwarts your efforts to help. You may feel frustrated at being unable to balance other aspects of your life with the burden of caregiving, especially if others are unhelpful. In a myriad of different ways, it may all seem "unfair." Excessive anger hurts your liver energy, and can create disharmony with the spleen and become depression. Master Nan Lu and Schaplowsky (2000, p.76) recommend throwing eggs at a tree to discharge anger—sure, laugh, but it works! Or practice the healing sounds of the tiger!

**JOY:** (See page 18). Having to give up time and energy when you have other tasks to manage may rob you of joy and bring about manic feelings in an attempt to get everything done. Excessive heart energy results in agitation. Agitation results from the disharmony between your kidney and heart. Practice the healing laughing sounds of a monkey to regain balance.

**WORRY:** Worry stems from a persistent feeling that the care you are providing is not good enough. You may feel that more must be done, or you may find yourself sweating about every little detail of caregiving. Ask yourself if all the little worries keep you from dealing with the one really big worry, i.e., the person you're caring for has dementia, is declining, and will eventually die. Exessive worry brings about anxiety. Recent research indicates that worrying may contribute to the development of Alzheimer's— for your sake, find a way to let it go. Raise your arms like a bear and ROAR from your belly. LET IT GO, let it go, let it go.

**GRIEF:** The essence of grief is loss. You may be anticipating a painful separation or even feelings of abandonment. You may be grieving because the hopes and plans you had for yourself (and others) may now be slipping away, or may even be unattainable. Excessive crying can damage the lungs. Release by practicing the healing sounds of a bird.

**FEAR:** You may fear that the situation will get worse or be out of your control. You may fear that you will run out of money, or that your loved one will die and you won't know what to do. Or you may fear that you, too, may die or have to abandon the person you are caring for. Guilt may set in from any or all of these emotions. Fear comes from the kidney. Imitate the sounds and movements of a deer.

---

According to caregiver.com (Seligson 1995–2013), burnout is "not like a cold" that passes relatively quickly. One may not even be aware of it at the time. But the "symptoms of burnout can surface months after a traumatic episode" and resemble post-traumatic stress disorder. Signs of burnout can range from fatigue and depression to withdrawal from social contacts, feelings of helplessness and an increasing fear of death. One Qigong student, who was the sole caregiver for her father, commented on the stark reality that some providers face:

> From my experience with Alzheimer's patients, they don't die from it as much as it "kills" the caregivers. It's taken me three years to recover from taking care of my dad. If I hadn't found this Qigong program last year, I don't think I would have recovered.

Because people with dementia often have bottled up emotions that cannot find adequate expression, caregivers know that it would be cruel to berate them for behaviors that can't be controlled, even though the caregiver might feel the impulse to do so. Moreover, conflicts can erupt when a person with memory loss accuses a caregiver of deceit or lying. Even though Ethleen had handed over financial responsibility to her daughter, she accused Lois of stealing money from her checkbook; similarly, Beverly accused her husband of seeing other women, even though he was with her "24/7." People identified as being in the middle stages of dementia —who have trouble recognizing their surroundings, family members or caregivers, or forget how to perform simple tasks like dressing—may also accuse others of things like stealing or infidelity. When there is an imagined sense of betrayal or some other wrongdoing, it is recommended that caregivers and family members refrain from arguing about what is imagined versus what is real. To the person experiencing memory loss, their emotions are real. Here's an example:

**Dad:** You stole my chocolate…my ice cream.

**Son:** No, I didn't. You ate the last of it yesterday. Remember? [Of course, he doesn't remember.]

**Dad** (louder): You stole my chocolate!

**Son:** How could I steal your ice cream when you ate it yesterday?

**Dad** (yelling): You stole it!

Okay, that didn't work out very well. Arguing in a legalistic way with people experiencing memory loss can be futile. Also, try not to use words like "remember." Even though a person with dementia may be incapable of verbalizing their shame at not being able to remember things, they may still feel it at some level; and that in turn may affect their behavior. Responding in a way that acknowledges the feelings, rather than the facts, makes it more likely that the person who has forgotten a recent event will move on. Let's try again, this time calmer:

**Dad:** You stole my chocolate...my ice cream.

**Son:** Geez, Dad, you seem upset. [Walking over to the refrigerator:] Oh look, there's some yummy pie—want some?

Dad looks around, a little confused, then smiles and shuffles toward the fridge, holding out his hands in anticipation. Balance is restored.

One of the most challenging aspects for a caregiver or family member is how to avoid taking verbal or physical aggression personally. This also applies to when the person with waning memory does not recognize a close relative or friend. Few emotions compare to the sinking feeling of hearing a loved one say, "Who are you?"

Here are some guidelines:

- **Read the need.** For the caregiver, the needs and afflictive emotions of the person under care can be very challenging. Moreover, the difficulties that caregivers face may be multi-determined, such as balancing the needs of career or other family members with the demands of caregiving. Ascertain where the source of discomfort is coming from; common grievances include fatigue, worry, or depression (including feelings of hopelessness and lack of control). In an effort to bring ease to the person being cared for, caregivers sometimes overlook their own health and wellbeing. If you are a caregiver, make sure that you are in touch with your own needs.

- **Address the need.** This can be challenging. In Beverly's case, Maura could have misread her mother's need during times of personal grooming and become engaged in the conflict. But by walking away, Maura gratified her mother's real need—to work it out by herself and thereby feel a sense of independence and control over her own life. Caregivers are encouraged to allow those under their care to do as much for themselves as possible, within the limits of safety and common sense. And by not "hovering," caregivers can find moments of peace and rest for themselves. Flexibility is key because conditions may change and require a different approach. If you are a caregiver, ensure that you are doing everything to take care of yourself.

- **Don't take it personally.** This can be particularly difficult for family members who have a history of conflict. Beverly's response to her mother being "feisty" is a good model for others. A short time-out for yourself can lessen the sting of conflict and do a world of good for all involved.

- **Change the setting or environment.** When working long hours, taking responsibility for others, or dealing with the unpredictable behaviors of people with dementia, a calmer setting is recommended. Some people may want to take a nap, listen to relaxing music, or meditate. Conversely, more stimulation may be needed: caregivers may enjoy singing, taking a stroll through the park, or catching a movie with a friend; interaction with others, especially children or friendly pets, can be very therapeutic.

- **Qigong.** Even simple movements like the Natural Healing Exercises for Hands and Feet in Part II can have a calming effect. Or, the caregiver and person experiencing memory lapses may need to vent their spleens (literally, from an energetic point of view) by releasing emotions through the Five Animal Forms, also in Part II. These exercises can help release pent-up emotions—anger, agitation, worry, grief, and fear—and common side effects of this practice may include smiles, laughter, and contentment. For individuals experiencing levels of stress, but not signs of dementia, negative emotions in the form of excess yin energy can impair organ functioning and create illness. An NHRF coach taught us how to help caregivers release pent up feelings by using a Heng-Ha exercise to discharge the excess yin energy. He also provided two meditations (sitting and lying down) at the end of this chapter that may help caregivers cultivate vital energy, lessen caustic inflammation, and restore their sense of calm and wellbeing. Finally, practicing the Twelve Sitting Exercises in Part II can build peace of mind through meditative movements.

In Chapter 3 the experience of a devoted caregiver, Maura, was presented as an example of someone who is caring for both of her parents. Her story is similar in many ways to people described as the "sandwich generation"—those taking care of their parents as well as their own children—since she is also busy raising a teenage daughter. But what seems to distinguish Maura from many caregivers is the absence of caregiver burnout, the all-too-common hazard of extended self-sacrifice; instead, she approaches her role with sparkling eyes, glowing skin, and an abundance of playful energy. This may be due in part to the fact that she not only guides her parents through natural healing exercises, but also practices with them. There is mounting evidence for the effectiveness of combining Western medicine and natural healing for those with symptoms of dementia and their caregivers.

For example, a study performed in 2013 called PLIÉ (Preventing Loss of Independence through Exercise) addressed the needs of both patients with dementia and their caregivers. The program demonstrated that a variety of exercises done regularly by seniors with dementia and their caregivers combined "the best of eastern and western exercise traditions" and improved outcomes for both.

---

A pilot study showed the program, which integrates functional movement and mindful body awareness, improved patients' cognitive and physical function and quality of life and reduced caregiver burden compared with usual care.

"This very small pilot study provides preliminary evidence [this program] may improve cognitive function, quality of life, physical function and caregiver burden with effect sizes that are substantially larger than what is typically seen with currently available dementia medications," principal investigator Deborah E. Barnes, PhD, MPH, University of California, San Francisco, and the San Francisco Veterans Affairs Medical Center, told delegates here attending the American Academy of Neurology 65th Annual Meeting.

Known as Preventing Loss of Independence through Exercise (PLIÉ), the program "combines the best elements of eastern and western exercise traditions including yoga, T'ai Chi, Feldenkrais, physical therapy, occupational therapy, mindfulness, and dance movement therapy," said Dr. Barnes (Cassels 2013).

---

As with people with dementia, it is essential for caregivers to find a way to release emotions that can mar their sense of wellbeing and, from the TCM perspective, damage their organ energy over time. It has been demonstrated that the smooth flow of energy through the meridians and organs promotes the functional interdependence and wellbeing of the entire system, which in turn releases afflictive emotions. Wouldn't it be great, then, if there was some special exercise that a caregiver and person with dementia symptoms could do together, that would be easy enough to be performed by someone limited by their decline, yet profound enough to release the pent-up emotions of both—and fun, too?

Yes, it would be great, and there is such an exercise, which, for want of a better name, could whimsically be called "Tigers and Monkeys and Bears—Oh my!" At the Qi Center in Hawaii strange animal sounds—the collective growl of seniors bellowing "GRRRRRR"—can be heard roaring from the practice room, rattling the bones. At that moment the seniors are imitating the sounds and body language of a tiger, enabling them to take on the personalities of that animal. Grandmaster developed a series of exercises for seniors and children, known as the Five Animal Forms, which combine the ancient practices of Healing Sounds and the Five Animal Frolics. These exercises imitate animal sounds and their energetic resonance to release afflictive emotions. Certain animals are associated with specific organs; for instance, the angry alcoholic who was mentioned earlier could practice the healing sound of the tiger— "GRRRRR"—to release anger from the liver.

Whether the emotional release can be attributed to psychological factors or the energetic release of stagnant Qi from an organ, it is worth reiterating that an "enriched environment" is optimal for those with memory impairment and their caregivers alike, for "maintaining the health of neurons, constructing synaptic connections, and building arterial highways to supply more blood to the brain" (World Tai Chi and Qigong Day 2005).

More evidence for the healing power of sounds comes from a 2011 study from researchers in New South Wales, who noted that roughly 75 percent of people with dementia experience "anxiety, distress or agitation." In a first-of-its-kind study on the effects of laugher on mood, researchers determined both short-term and long-term benefits to participants from laughter therapy, but without the side effects of antipsychotic drugs.

> The researchers found that the humor intervention worked well for almost all the patients. The laughter therapy also minimized the potential for such risks as falling and premature death often associated with prescription meds. In all, the researchers calculated a 20 percent drop in overall agitation. And this decrease lasted for at least 14 weeks beyond the conclusion of the program.
>
> (The Doctors Health Press 2011b)

Since Marcia began teaching the Five Animal Forms and other exercises from the Senior Wellness Program, she has witnessed similar changes to those experienced by the seniors taught by the NHRF Coordinator of the Senior classes and other volunteers. The class members engage physically and emotionally to the point where their once dull emotions transformed into the enthusiastic growls, laughter, and roars of the animal sounds. Many residents remember these exercises from week to week and request to participate in that activity over other choices. In one instance, a married man joined his wife for the first time in an activity; in another, a woman who used to sit completely withdrawn began to wave her hands like a conductor to the accompanying music and participate in the healing sounds portion of the exercises.

For people with indicators of dementia and caregivers alike, the series of chair exercises presented in Part II of this book will help them to feel that each day they are coming a little more alive.

## Heng-Ha Exercise

This exercise is only for those individuals who have no indications of memory loss. The responsibility of ministering to the needs of others can impose overwhelming pressures that, if left untreated, can bring about illness and burnout. Therefore, the need for caregivers to release pent-up emotions is so important that a simple exercise has been included here to help providers restore their sense of calm and wellbeing. There are many useful exercises to relieve stress, but the Heng-Ha exercise from the NHRF is particularly recommended because of its effectiveness in applying just two distinctive sounds during movement to release afflictive emotions from the body and restore balance in the energetic system.

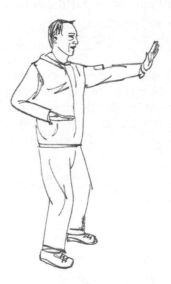

*Figure 4.1 Heng-Ha stance.*

## *Heng-Ha Exercise for Caregivers*
**Guidelines:**

- Stand with your legs shoulder-width apart and knees slightly bent.

- Extend your left arm straight out in front of you, hand pulled back with fingers pointing toward the ceiling like you're saying, "Stop!"

- Pull the right hand back toward the armpit, palm facing up, and fingers pointing straight forward.

- Rapidly switch hand positions. Push the right hand forward and rotate the palm facing up with the fingers pointing toward the ceiling as you simultaneously withdraw the left hand back to your ribs with the palm facing up and fingers pointing forward. As you push the right hand forward, forcefully expel your breath with a "Heng" sound.

- Then, as you thrust your left hand forward while simultaneously withdrawing your right hand, forcefully expel your breath with a "Ha" sound.

- Repeat these thrusting and withdrawing movements with their respective sounds until you feel calm and energized. Take care not to overdo this exercise, as you might expend too much energy and feel more tired.

## The Miracle of Meditation

Throughout the world, millions of people practice meditation daily. Research now confirms what individuals who are proficient in Qigong, Yoga, and other spiritual traditions have observed empirically for thousands of years. Meditation activates the parasympathetic response and confers benefits that include the following: abatement in cortisol and the inflammatory response, as well as reductions in disorders such as insomnia, anxiety and depression; increase in blood levels of endorphins and the immune response; and activation in "frontal and subcortical brain regions" that are important for "sustained attention and emotion regulation." (Semel Institute 2013) These restorative effects are an essential tool for caregivers, as shown by a recent study conducted at UCLA that brings hope to caregivers who are overwhelmed and experiencing mental and physical distress:

Our recently published brief daily yogic meditation (Kirtan Kriya) for stressed family dementia caregivers with mild depressive symptoms found that meditation resulted in lower levels of depressive symptoms, as well as improvements in mental health and cognitive functioning. Participants in the yogic meditation group showed a 43 percent improvement in telomerase activity after 12 minutes of daily practice for 8 weeks, compared with 3.7

percent in relaxation music control participants. This suggests that brief daily meditation practices can not only lead to improved mental and cognitive functioning, but may also benefit stress-induced cellular aging.

(Semel Institute 2013)

As we have seen, the constant stress of supportive care can impair caregivers' health over time. The Five Element Theory explains one important aspect of an individual's declining health and vitality in terms of an excess or deficiency of Mind, which restrains the life force, Qi. The magic of meditation, then, resides in its ability to ease thinking and thus activate the flow of vital energy throughout the energetic system. Hence, beginners of meditation will commonly describe tickling or itchy sensations on the face. This signals that vital energy is beginning to flow through the meridians of the face with a resultant rush of blood into the capillaries. Over time people who meditate note additional sensations that follow a predictable course and reach ever deeper levels of the body, including the organs and bones. As channels remain open, some of these sensations become less palpable while the benefits become more pronounced.

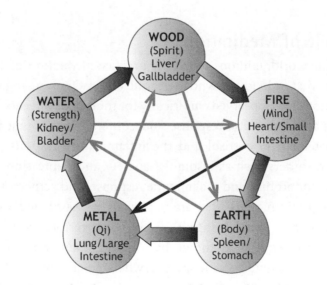

*Figure 4.2. In this chart, an excess or deficiency of Mind restrains Qi. Vital energy flows better when the mind and body are relaxed, so practices that quiet the mind promote the flow of Qi.*

## *Self-Healing Meditation for Caregivers*

For thousands of years in China, the practice of Qigong has taught many different meditation techniques: posture—standing, sitting, or lying down; changes in breathing during inhale and exhale, reverse breathing; Mudras (hand positions), and more; but, the essence of meditation for cultivating energy—with its many benefits—typically combines the same principles, which are easy to do.

### Getting started

- Sit comfortably on a chair with your feet flat on the floor.

- Use a pillow under your "sit bones" if needed to bring your hips up a little to be level with or higher than your knees.

- Roll your shoulders back in a circle once or twice to help make your spine straight and relaxed.

- Place your hands on your lap near your body, one hand over the other with your palms facing up. Women put their right hand on top, men their left hand; tips of thumbs touching.

- In the beginning, meditate for only a few minutes and then try for longer. Over time you will naturally meditate longer.

## *Daily Meditation for Relaxation (sitting)*

- Sit with your back in a posture that is straight but not rigid.

- Let the tip of your tongue rest naturally on the roof of your mouth.

- Gently close your mouth and smile. It will relax your face and head, and it will open energy pathways.

- Let out a long exhale to quiet your mind and continue with slow, abdominal breathing. During the exhale breathe relaxation into your pelvic region and then down to the feet. Let your mind rest in a space of awareness without thinking, empty and free.

## Daily Meditation for Deeper Sleep (lying down)

- To begin, lie down in bed on your back. Rest your tongue comfortably on the roof of your mouth and breathe from your abdomen. During the exhale breathe relaxation into your pelvic region and then down to the feet.

- Slowly curl and uncurl your fingers, fanning your fingers out as you uncurl them. Be gentle, using no tension.

- Then place your hands beside you on the bed and focus on your feet.

- Gently curl and uncurl your toes several times, fanning them out as you uncurl them.

- Hold your toes lightly curled until you feel like letting go. Ease into sleep and wake up feeling rejuvenated!

## Meditation Reminders for Gathering Energy

The practice of meditation requires patience and commitment to accumulate Qi. Here are a few helpful reminders for your daily meditation.

When you place the tip of your tongue on the roof of your mouth, it completes a circuit of two major channels of energy. Over time the tongue will naturally connect with the roof of your mouth.

In the Five Element Theory, an excess of Mind restrains Qi (see page 62). If your mind begins to wander or jump around with incessant chatter ("monkey brain"), simply bring your attention back to your breathing.

The natural length of your meditation should be based upon how alert you feel. If you are having trouble maintaining your posture, feel mentally tired, or are about to fall asleep, it is time to stop meditating. Know that even brief meditations throughout the day can enhance your wellbeing. Over time, you will find that the duration of your meditation will increase naturally and that you will feel more energetic and vital throughout the day.

Do not try to force gathering energy or move it before its natural time. If you wish to cultivate meditations longer than 20 minutes, consult with a trained teacher of meditation for supervision.

# 5

# Conclusion to Part I

If there is one concept that Qigong emphasizes time and time again, it is that humans are intimately, if not inextricably, linked with the universe. One way to think about it is that the little universe of our bodies is connected energetically with cycles of energy in the big universe. This can be experienced inside of us through occurrences such as seasons, time of day, weather, and tides, to name a few.

Through your own Qigong practice, self-healing, and study, you can discover these energetic connections with the outer world. Energy travels through all living things, connecting all living things together. To harness this energy through natural healing and rejuvenate people with all forms of dementia, it helps to understand how we are connected to the bigger universe.

People sensitive to the flow of energy—masters of Qigong, T'ai Chi, and Yoga—can tell time just by the feel of energetic sensations in their bodies. For example, if the sensations of tingling or "bubbling" are felt prominently on the soles of their feet between the second and third metatarsals, they will know that the time of day falls between 5:00 p.m. and 7:00 p.m. This spot is the beginning of the kidney meridian on the acupuncture chart and is called Bubbling Well. It flows there most strongly during the time of day when energy courses through the kidney channel, and it is passing through members of their family and neighbors at that moment, too; it is flowing through the kidney channels of their pets—dogs, cats, and parakeets—as well as the mice in the basement. It is flowing in the park, through the ducks in the pond and through the squirrels at the picnic tables. It is flowing through the kidney channels of all living things in that time zone. Where blockages develop in this system, for creatures big and small, problems arise in the kidney energy that affects other organs related to kidney functioning.

For people with dementia like Ethleen and Jane, this connection with the larger picture could be seen through their emotions of fear and agitation, which became particularly acute toward evening during the time known for sundowning. Kidneys, undernourished of vital energy during what might be thought of as their feeding time, act out with behaviours of fear: panic, confusion, agitation, trembling, cold extremities, or an urgent need to use the bathroom. Natural healing believes that much of this distress can be eased through exercises that simply restore the flow of vital energy.

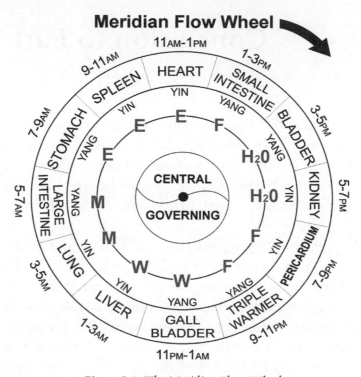

*Figure 5.1. The Meridian Flow Wheel.*

The Meridian Flow Wheel (Poole 2008) illustrates the times during a 24-hour cycle when the vital energy emanating from the "big universe" courses, like ocean tides, through the "little universe" of our bodies. We receive this Qi in the form of two opposite and complementary energies, yin and yang. In the Introduction we also noted the circular nature of the yin–yang symbol, which indicates that the two energies are interdependent and that each contains a part of the opposite within it.

Qigong practice reveals yin–yang pairs and can readily be felt during exercises, such as the sequence known as Gather the Energy Ball (see Awakening Healing Energy in Part II). As you rub your hands together to generate heat and then pull them apart with fingers curled, you can sense the expanding and contracting energies of yin and yang, like an invisible ball between your hands. At that point the yin–yang symbol is no longer a mere philosophical construct or trendy ornament hanging from a car mirror. Instead, it becomes known and experienced as a universal principle.

In the human body, organs are either yin or yang and function as complementary pairs. For instance, the kidney is yin and its paired organ, the bladder, is yang. These pairs are also energetically interconnected with other organ pairs through the meridians—like sprinklers connected through underground pipes—so that no organ functions exclusive of the others. This knowledge is one of the great gifts of TCM because it describes how diseases like dementia can originate from the stagnation of energy in the organs, not just from an illness in the brain. For a person showing indications of dementia, this supports the possibility of both early detection and the improvement of health.

The Five Element Theory is used in this book to describe organs and their connection to the basic components of nature, as well as the manner in which they function within our bodies: for example, we have seen how the kidney (water) promotes the liver (wood), just as rain nourishes a tree; yet, when unbalanced, it restrains the heart (fire), just as water douses a flame. You might wonder if this is substantiated by what is known in Western medicine. Yes: diseases of the kidney cause high blood pressure, which can then damage the heart.

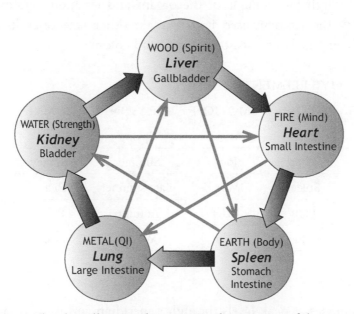

*Figure 5.2. This chart illustrates the way yin and yang organs of the Five Elements complement and promote each other. However, same pair organs, like yang/yang organs or the yin/yin organs dealt with in this book—liver, heart, spleen, lung and kidney—will restrain one another if there is an imbalance in the system.*

As one becomes familiar with this conceptualization, aspects of our everyday experience, including health and psychology, crystallize in ways where connections did not previously seem to exist. Someone who "thinks too much" (excess of Mind) restrains Qi that nourishes the body. Conversely, an athletic person with a superior IQ might nevertheless experience an inability to "think clearly" during times of overexertion and could inappropriately be labeled by others as having "more brawn than brains."

In previous chapters we noted how afflictive emotions are tied to organ energy that is blocked or by the restraint of energy from another organ; for example, for those experiencing indications of dementia, a deficiency of Qi in the kidney restrains the heart and may provoke sundown syndrome. This example highlights the interdependence of organs and the need for balancing energy throughout the system. In the larger sense, we can also see a functional interdependence among people, such as exists between a caregiver and a person with dementia. The two form yin–yang pairs, just as people do in everyday interactions such as friendships, sports, lovemaking, and politics. These are not static relationships but relative ones, in which the roles can evolve and change. When the yin and yang of the pair change in disproportionate ways, the energies become imbalanced and dysfunction can follow.

Now that we have seen how the "little universe" connects with the "big universe" through the example of the organs and emotions, we can further explore how the Chinese used it to explain other categories in The Five Element Theory, including season, animal, and color.

## TABLE 5.1. FIVE ELEMENTS THEORY

| ELEMENT | ORGAN | EMOTION | SEASON | ANIMAL | COLOR |
|---------|-------|---------|--------|--------|-------|
| **WOOD** | Liver | Anger | Spring | Tiger | Green |
| **FIRE** | Heart | Joy* | Summer | Monkey | Red |
| **EARTH** | Spleen | Worry | Late summer | Bear | Yellow |
| **METAL** | Lung | Grief | Autumn | Bird | White |
| **WATER** | Kidney | Fear | Winter | Deer | Dark blue |

* See Joy, page 18.

Just as Qi courses at peak levels through a meridian and its associated organ during a specific time of day, organs are nurtured more favourably during specific seasons of the year. A dynamic stability between the organs is what can create optimal health; but when the energies of the organs are out of balance, dysfunction can ensue. The liver, for example, is the organ of spring and is associated with the element of wood. In the promotional cycle, kidney energy promotes the liver; or, in the language of the Five Element Theory (see Figure 5.1), the water of kidneys promotes the wood of liver. Like dominos falling, if the liver is not functioning properly, it restrains the spleen, causing the spleen to overproduce phlegm that clogs the lungs. So people who have allergies brought on by pollens during springtime may lessen or eliminate their symptoms by ensuring that their kidneys are well nourished during the winter months (Lui and Gong 2009). The Western model is to stabilize the dysfunction in the body with the use of antihistamines, decongestants, and nasal corticosteroids. However, Morelli and Chang (2014) list a variety of common side effects that range from fast heartbeat and increased blood pressure to nervousness, stomach problems, and trouble sleeping.

The current medications for people diagnosed with dementia can likewise carry serious side effects, which is why the FDA requires "boxed warnings" for atypical antipsychotic medications used in the treatment of behavioral issues associated with dementia (Doctor's Health Press Editorial Board 2005). By contrast, natural healing works to reduce the stagnation of Qi and disharmonies in the energetic system in order to strengthen organ energy. A famous Tao Master, Shen Chia-Shu, in the Ching dynasty addressed concerns about medications that still resonate today: "Breathing and related exercises are one hundred times more effective as medical therapy than any drug."

Another oft cited category in the Five Element Theory is animal. There are five animals—tiger, monkey, bear, bird, and deer—associated with the five pairs of the vital organs in the body. The movements and sounds of these animals are imitated to stimulate the energy of each organ pair, thereby clearing blockages, releasing afflictive emotions, and allowing vital Qi to flow through newly opened channels. While sound therapy is a very ancient method of healing, it is fun to perform and can easily be integrated into Western practices for improved health. The exercises for this Qigong practice will be described in Part II, Chapter 7.

Although there are many more categories associated with the Five Element Theory, the final one offered here is the relationship between color and food. Ask yourself these questions: What are three foods that are recommended for your heart? And what do they have in common? A typical answer might be watermelon, tomatoes, and cranberries. In common, these foods and "other red fruits and vegetables, such as strawberries, raspberries, and beets contain anthocyanins (pronounced an-tho-SIGH-uh-nins), a group of phytochemicals that are powerful antioxidants that help control high blood pressure and protect against diabetes-related circulatory problems" (Wiley's Supper Club 2014). Other health benefits include scrubbing free radicals from the body, protecting eye health, and reducing the chance of developing prostate cancer, to name a few. But mainly, these foods are highly recommended for protecting the heart and—from a TCM point of view—it is significant that they are all the color red. So are goji berries and red dates, which similarly protect the heart. Amazing as it may sound to a Western sensibility, TCM demonstrates that when you match the color of a food with the organ it represents, the essence of the food has a property that addresses the specific needs of the organ's energy. Looking at the color of foods through the lens of TCM, then, you begin to see their properties from a "big universe" perspective. The proof in the "little universe" comes from the enhanced health these foods provide.

For people experiencing any type of memory loss, the NHRF recommends foods that address the root cause of dementia: low kidney energy. As we saw in Chapter 1, low kidney energy affects the bones and bone marrow. When red blood cell production from the bone marrow is diminished, the brain can't get the oxygen it needs, which reduces kidney energy even more. For natural healing, foods are suggested that are high in protein, fiber, and vitamins, including the following: whole grains (brown rice, barley), vegetables (celery, lily flower, and eggplant), black mushrooms, roasted nuts (macadamia, walnuts, and hazelnuts), and seeds (black sesame seeds, pine nuts, and buckwheat). It is important to note that many of these foods are predominantly dark, the color for the kidney (see Part III, "Foods to Awaken Natural Healing").

Many of the foods for natural healing also contain high levels of omega-3 fatty acids vitamins, and phytonutrients, which are shown to have properties that counteract the corrosive effects that lead to nerve damage and dementia:

> Nerve cells in the brain are networked and organized to perform various different tasks. Chronic oxidative and inflammatory stress can progressively damage those nerve cells as well as organized networks causing Alzheimer's disease. Therefore, food with anti-oxidative and anti-inflammatory effects may have a potential in preventing such nerve damage. (Shah 2013)

Walnuts in particular are a rich source of omega-3 fatty acids, which, according to Dr. Frank Sacks at the Department of Nutrition, Harvard School of Public Health, "confer potential benefits for a wide range of conditions," including protection against heart disease, cancer, and autoimmune diseases, to name a few. He concludes that foods rich in omega-3 fatty acids contain essential nutrients for wellbeing:

> For good health, you should aim to get at least one rich source of omega-3 fatty acids in your diet every day. This could be through a serving of fatty fish (such as salmon), a tablespoon of canola or soybean oil in salad dressing or in cooking, or a handful of walnuts or ground flaxseed mixed into your morning oatmeal. (Sacks 2014)

At the beginning of this book I asked: What is the essence of natural healing and where can it be found? If nothing else, I hope this book has helped the reader understand that the essence resides within the little universe of our bodies and is energetically coupled with the big universe. Once that is grasped, it is only a matter of finding the means to mobilize the natural healing within. The mind–body connection is just beginning to be understood by Western medicine (for example, in stress and migraine headaches); but the Chinese have known for thousands of years how to release the stresses and traumas that become imbedded in our tissues and contribute to ongoing physical and emotional distress. So much depends upon simply changing our minds and then making sensible changes that will enhance the flow of energy in ourselves, or in someone we care about.

People who practice Qigong usually seek to dwell in a state of balance in their everyday lives, which is represented in the yin–yang symbol by the line that separates the two. By living in a state of balance—not too yin, not too yang—it is possible to better manage the ups and downs that life brings. For caregivers, their functional interdependence with someone with dementia necessitates a working understanding of this; metaphorically, they have to keep their feet rooted to the deck, and their bodies strong yet flexible as their boat pitches on a roiling sea; when becalmed, they have to row.

It is the hope of everyone who has contributed to this book that we have shed a new light on the process of dementia, with keys to unlocking the body's ability to rejuvenate itself where possible. *Qigong for Wellbeing in Dementia and Aging* is not just for the person experiencing symptoms of dementia, but also for anyone concerned with the disease. Throughout Part I it has been shown that memory loss is not just a decline in brain functioning but also a systemic decline in organ energy. In this regard the practices in Part II will help to clear disharmonies throughout the body and can be practiced by anyone for overall fitness—not least as part of a comprehensive health care plan. While this book's primary purpose is to introduce simple and easy natural healing principles and exercises, we have included a comprehensive listing of resources if you would like to explore in greater depth the rich history, practice, and efficacy of Qigong.

*After about a year of Qigong, I have never felt so good as I do now. I could barely lift my hands up to my head area. Now I can slowly inch my way to the sides of my head, past my ears, and I don't get sick anymore.*

80-year-old man

Part II of this book, "Exercises to Awaken Natural Healing," presents a program of Qigong exercises that were developed by the NHRF to benefit seniors and the aging brain. The program includes hand and feet exercises, animal sounds, facial massages and 12 Sitting Exercises for movement and meditation. In applying the natural healing program for someone who is showing indications of dementia, or as a preventative practice for people concerned about their own memory, results may be seen that offer a complement to an existing health program. Whether for yourself or someone you care about, natural healing can offer an improved sense of wellbeing.

To start, practice as many of the exercises in Part II as you can while sitting comfortably in a chair, preferably one with arms. Add more repetitions and exercises as comfort allows. When bending or stretching, raising your arms, or stretching your feet, go only as far as the body comfortably allows. Over time, the range of motion should increase naturally so it will feel better to do more.

The recommendations in this book need to be discussed with your doctor. Always check to see if this program is suitable for you, or someone under your care, before using the natural healing suggestions in this book. If you are sick or weak, you need to see your doctor because this program is not a medical treatment.

# PART II

## Exercises to Awaken
## NATURAL HEALING

# 6

# Natural Healing Exercises Using the Hands and Feet
## Contributed by the Natural Healing Research Foundation

Aging starts from the feet. Our feet are the farthest point of the body from the heart, central nervous system, internal organs, and major systems of the body. There is a close relationship between the brain, memory, and hands. The beginning and end points of all major meridians can be found on the hands and feet. Reflex points and reflex zones for all internal organs are distributed on the hands and feet. Therefore, exercises using the hands and feet work the extremities from a reverse direction to activate the circulatory, neural, and lymphatic systems of the body. These exercises are a simple and easy form of physical conditioning for the body. The hands and feet exercises are done while sitting in a chair, preferably one with arms, in whatever clothing you happen to be wearing.

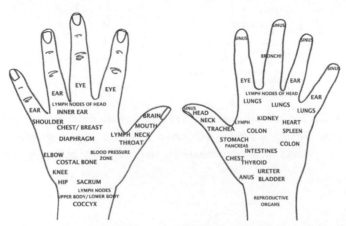

*Figure 6.1. The hand is dotted with many reflexology points, both on the top of the hand and on the palm. Massaging these point areas on the hands and doing hand exercises stimulates a good flow of energy, blood, and oxygen to promote the energy of each organ.*

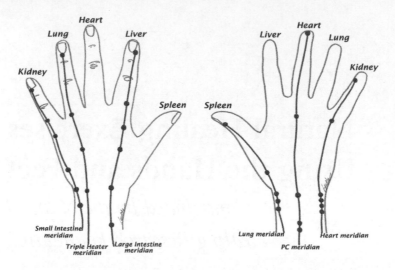

*Figure 6.2. When there are excesses or deficiencies in the energies of the internal organs, those imbalances manifest physically on the fingers and toes. The characteristic of each toe or finger — its shape, skin color, and relative proportions —represent the condition of the organ to which it relates. Those specific characteristics provide a glimpse into the wellbeing of each organ.*

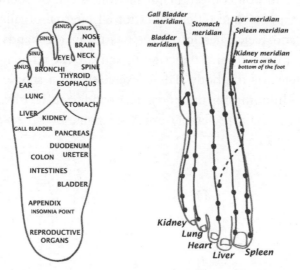

*Figure 6.3. Meridian channels for some organs run through the hands and feet also. Massaging points along these channels and doing hand and feet exercises helps to stimulate the flow of blood and energy through the body and to the brain.*

# GATHER YOUR ENERGY AND GET IT MOVING WITH A SERIES OF NINE EXERCISES FOR THE HANDS

## 1. WARM UP YOUR ENERGY

1. Press your palms and fingers firmly together and rub up and down quickly until your hands and thumbs feel warm and tingly.

2. Then spread your fingers apart a little to rub the inside of your fingers.

3. Finish with your hands pressed together, fingers pointing up.

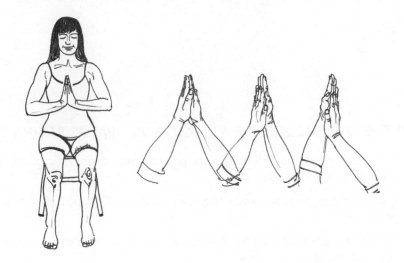

## 2. TAP YOUR FINGER TIPS TO AWAKEN YOUR ENERGY

1. Start with your warm hands pressed together and your fingers pointing up.

2. Pull your palms apart as you keep your fingertips pressing into each other.

3. Round your fingers and palms out until there is enough room to hold a ball. It may feel like you are holding a soft, warm ball of energy.

4. Keep your elbows down so your wrists do not bend.

5. Tap your finger and thumb tips together at least 12 times without losing the rounded shape of your fingers.

6. Tap at least 12 more times as you pull your hands farther apart, making your "energy ball" larger.

7. Tap at least 12 more times with your eyes closed as you bring your hands closer together.

8. Press your hands back together with your fingers pointing up.

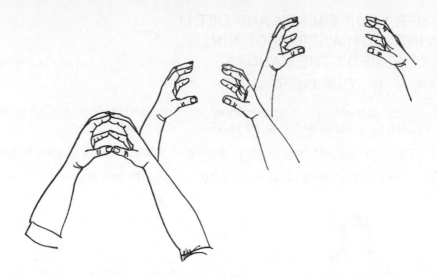

## 3. TAP THE OUTER EDGES OF YOUR HANDS—PALMS FACING YOU

1. With your palms together, fingers pointed up, open your hands like a book so your palms face you.

2. Tap the sides of your hands together at least 12 times at a moderate pace.

3. Continue tapping at least 12 more times as you stretch your arms straight out in front of you.

4. Tap at least 12 more times as you bring your hands back in front of you.

5. Close your palms back together to begin the next exercise.

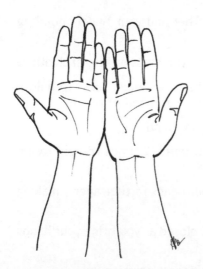

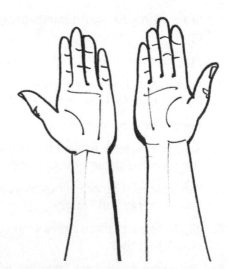

## 4. TAP THE INNER EDGES OF YOUR HANDS—PALMS FACING AWAY

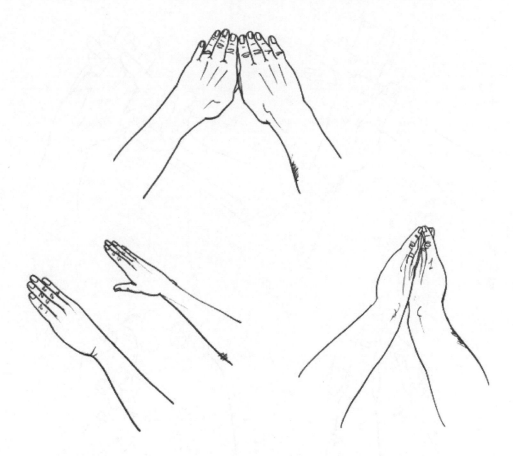

1.  With your palms together, fingers pointed up, open your hands so that the backs of your hands face you and the sides of your index fingers are touching. Your thumbs will be pointing out in front of your hands.

2.  Tap the sides of your index fingers together at least 12 times.

3.  Stretch your hands straight out in front of you as you tap at least 12 more times.

4.  Now roll your hands inwards so the backs of your hands are touching.

5.  Tap the backs of your hands, fingers and fingernails together at least 12 times.

6.  Now roll your hands back so your palms are facing the floor again.

7.  Tap the inside edges of your hands at least 12 times as you bring your hands back towards you.

8.  Roll your hands back together until your palms are fully touching and your fingers are pointing up.

## 5. RUBBING YOUR PALMS TO AWAKEN MORE ENERGY

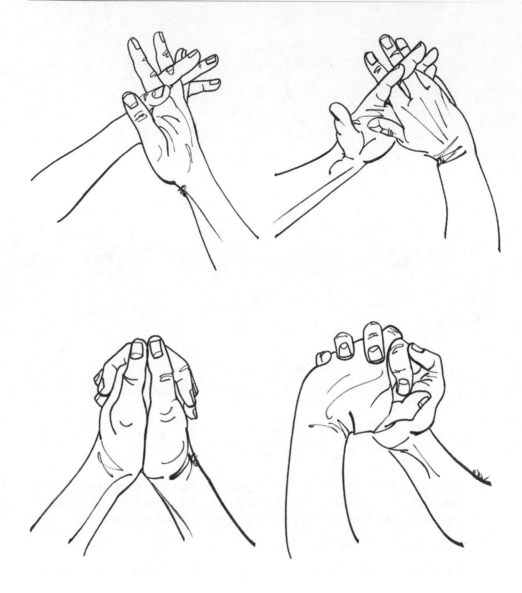

1.  Start with your palms pressed together in front of you, fingers pointed up.
2.  Slide your fingers between each other until you are pressing into your webs.
3.  Wiggle your hands and fingers back and forth and around to massage the webs of your fingers.

4.  Now grip your fingers completely onto the backs of your hands and tightly press the heels of your palms together.

5.  Rub the heels of your palms back and forth up to 24 times as your wrists twist to accommodate the motion.

6.  Without releasing your folded hands, lower your hands to your lap and let your palms face upward. Breathe peacefully for a minute or so.

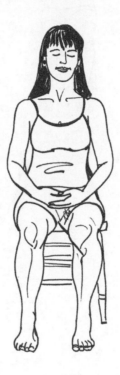

## 6. HAPPY BUDDHA STRETCHES YOUR ENERGY UP

1.  Relax your face by letting your tongue rest naturally on the roof of your mouth and gently smile during the entire exercise.

2.  Clasp your hands together on your lap with your palms facing up. Gaze at your clasped hands through all of this exercise.

3.  Raise your hands toward your face. As they reach your face, turn your hands so they are facing away from you and stretch them straight up above your head.

4.  Keep looking up with a smile. Pull your arms back as far as you can.

5.  Push against your fingers and then release your clasp.

6.  Let your hands and arms float down. Do this stretch up to eight times.

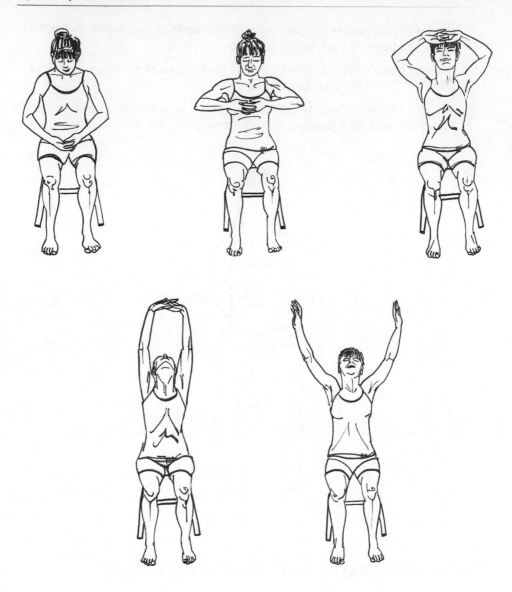

## 7. HAPPY BUDDHA STRETCHES YOUR ENERGY OUT

1. Relax your face by letting your tongue rest naturally on the roof of your mouth and gently smile during the entire exercise.

2. Clasp your hands together on your lap with your palms facing up. Gaze at your clasped hands through all of this exercise.

3. Bring your clasped hands up to chest level.

4. Rotate your hands until your palms face away from you.

5. Stretch your hands and arms straight out in front of you as far as you can stretch. Let your shoulders round a little to do this.

6.  Push against your fingers and then release your clasp.

7.  Let your hands float down. Do this stretch up to eight times.

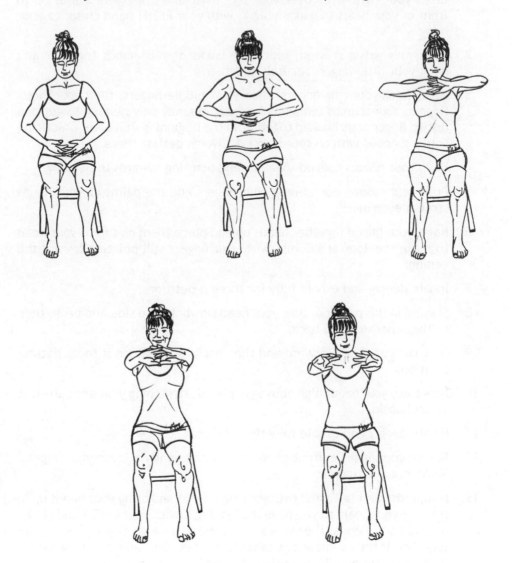

## 8. ROOSTER'S COMB FINGER AND HAND STRETCHES

1.  Cross your right wrist over your left wrist and bring your hands up in front of your heart to make a big X, with your RIGHT hand closer to your body.

2.  With your wrists crossed, touch the backs of your hands together and hook your little fingers securely together.

3.  Next, hook your ring fingers, then your middle fingers, then your index fingers. Your thumbs remain unhooked. You may only be able to get one or two finger pairs hooked together in the beginning, but after practicing you'll succeed with all four pairs! It's worth getting there.

4.  Keep your fingers hooked together and pointing towards the ceiling.

5.  Push your elbows out to help your fingers and the palms of your hands stretch even more.

6.  Raise your linked together hands up and place them on top of your head to make the Rooster's Comb, with your fingers still pointing toward the ceiling.

7.  Inhale deeply and exhale fully for three repetitions.

8.  Staying in this position, turn your head slowly to one side and back, then to the other side and back.

9.  Now tilt your head forward and then backward. Return it to its natural position.

10. Now raise your hands high above your head, stretching your arms straight up and back.

11. Inhale deeply and exhale fully three times.

12. Return your hands in front of your heart and gently release your fingers. Shake out your hands.

13. Now, cross your left wrist over your right wrist and bring your hands up in front of your heart so you have made a big X with your LEFT hand closer to your body. Repeat the same steps above to hook all of your finger pairs together. It is very important to do both sides. One side is usually harder than the other and it's important to give it practice, too.

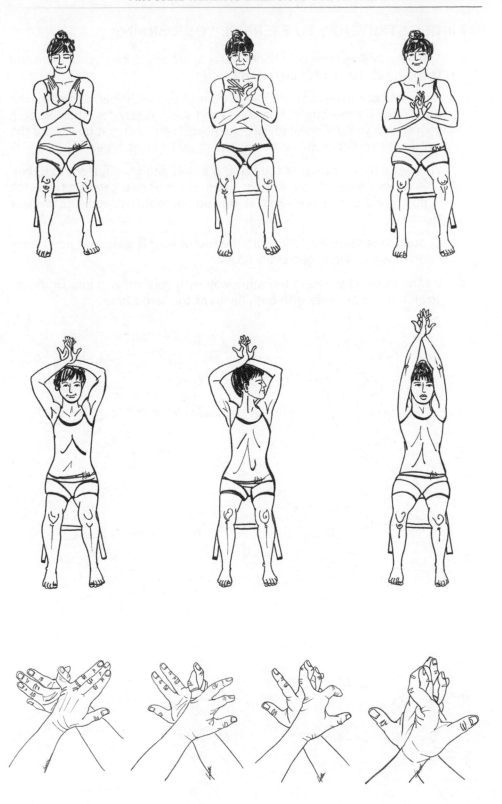

## 9. FINGER STRETCHES TO EXERCISE YOUR BRAIN

1.  Spread your fingers on both hands as far apart as you can, relax them and then repeat the stretch up to eight times.

2.  Now, hold one hand outstretched in front of you with your elbow relaxed (or resting on the arm of the chair) and your fingers together. Stretch your thumb straight down toward the floor. Then stretch it up toward the ceiling. Repeat this up-and-down stretch up to eight times.

3.  With your hand staying in the same position and your fingers together, stretch your index finger straight down as far as you can. Then stretch it up toward the ceiling. Repeat this up-and-down stretch up to eight times.

4.  Continue the same stretches with the rest of your fingers, one at a time—middle finger, ring finger, pinky finger.

5.  Do the same stretches in the same way with your other hand. Or, finger stretches can be done with both hands at the same time.

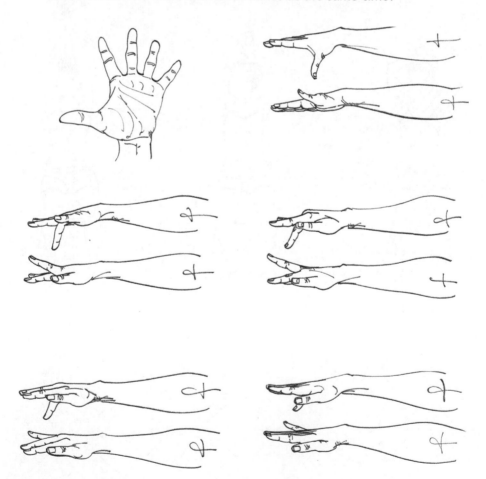

## STIMULATE FOOT ENERGY AND MOVE IT WITH A SERIES OF SIX EXERCISES FOR THE FEET

The Chinese say we age from the feet up, so don't miss doing these simple yet important exercises. They take five to six minutes to complete. These foot exercises are done while sitting comfortably in a chair.

### 1. POINT YOUR TOES TO GET YOUR ENERGY MOVING

1. Raise one foot off the floor.
2. Point your toes away from you for a count of two.
3. Pull your foot back toward you as much as you can for a count of two.
4. Do five or more sets of pointing.
5. Lower your foot to the floor and raise the other foot.
6. Repeat the above directions for the other foot.

As you pull your toes back, feel the stretch up the backs of your legs.

**Advanced practice:**

1. With both feet raised off the floor, alternate, with one foot pointing away from your body, as the other foot points toward your body.
2. Continue alternating back and forth, at least eight times.

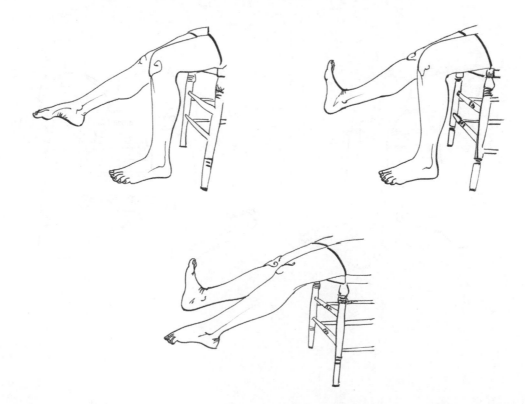

## 2. CIRCLE YOUR FEET TO CLEAR ENERGY PATHWAYS

1.  Start with your feet flat on the floor.

2.  Lift your lower legs and feet a few inches off the floor.

3.  Rotate your ankles around and around, so your feet make circles going in the same direction.

4.  Make at least five circles. More if you like.

5.  Now reverse and make at least five circles in the other direction.

6.  Rest your feet on the floor.

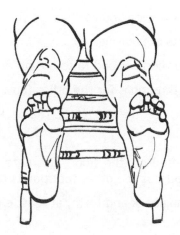

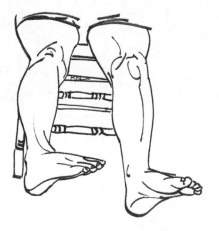 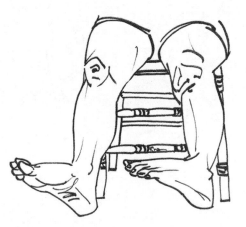

## 3. ROCK YOUR FEET TO MAKE ENERGY

1.  Start with your feet flat on the floor.

2.  Rock up onto the balls of your feet so that your heels are off the floor.

3.  Then rock back onto the heels of your feet, lifting the front of your feet off the floor.

4.  Repeat at least eight times.

**Advanced practice:**

1.  Alternate rocking your feet so that you're up on the ball of one foot while you're back on the heel of the other: heel and ball, ball and heel.

2.  Add in swinging your arms back and forth like you are walking.

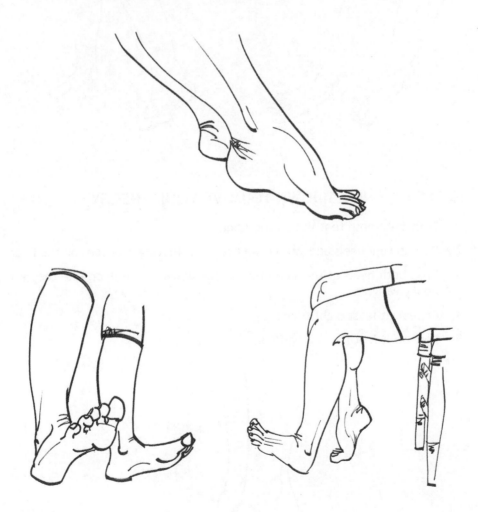

## 4. YIN-YANG FEET TO BALANCE YOUR ENERGY

1. Start with your feet flat on the floor.

2. Roll both of your feet to one side until you are resting on the side edges of both feet.

3. Then, roll both of your feet to the other side until you are resting on the opposite side edges of both feet.

4. Repeat rocking from side to side at least five complete times.

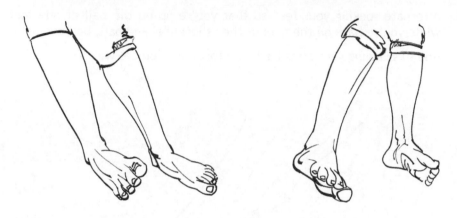

## 5. HEELS UP / HEELS DOWN TO MOVE YOUR ENERGY

1. Start with both feet flat on the floor.

2. Pick up your heels and stretch your feet up, leaving your toes on the floor.

3. Drop both heels at the same time, back down to the floor, like they are heavy weights.

4. Repeat at least eight times.

5. Rest both feet flat on the floor.

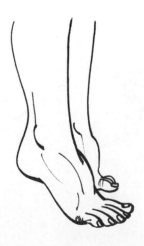

## 6. STOMP AND CLAP TO MOVE ENERGY THROUGHOUT YOUR BODY

1. Stomp each foot flat on the floor to a count of:

2. 1...2...3...4...1...2...3...4... Now faster: 1.2.3.4.1.2.3.4.

3. Clap your hands fully together to the count of:

4. 1...2...3...4...1...2...3...4... Now faster: 1.2.3.4.1.2.3.4.

5. Now STOMP and CLAP at the same time to the count of:

6. 1...2...3...4...1...2...3...4... Now faster: 1.2.3.4.1.2.3.4.

7. Stomp and clap for at least three complete sets.

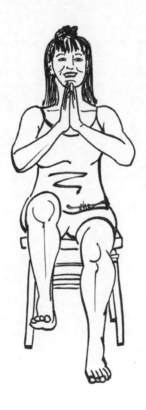 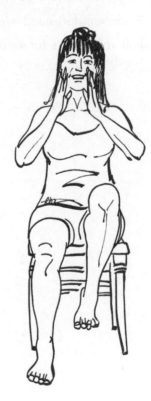

## CLOSING MEDITATION TO STORE THE ENERGY

**Men:**

- Place your left hand in the center of your lower abdomen, about three inches below your belly button.

- Place your right hand over your left hand.

- Roll your hands forward so your palms are facing up with your thumbs touching.

**Women:**

- Place your right hand in the center of your lower abdomen, about three inches below your belly button.

- Place your left hand over your right hand.

- Roll your hands forward so your palms are facing up with your thumbs touching.

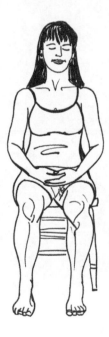

## The meditation

- Let your tongue rest naturally on the roof of your mouth.

- Relax your face into a smile.

- Deeply inhale and exhale from your abdomen at least three times.

# 7

# Releasing Harmful Emotions through the Five Animal Forms

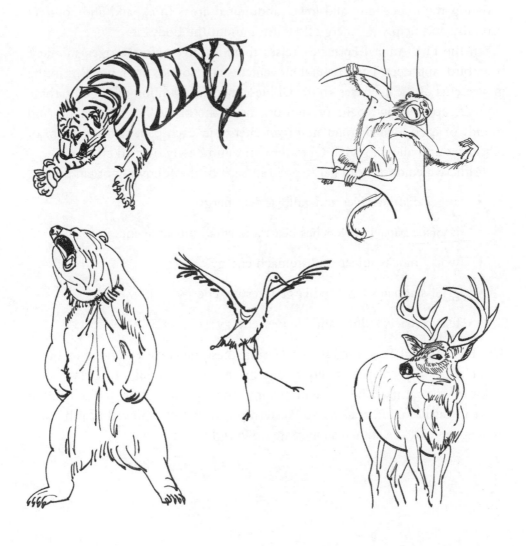

## Animal Sounds and Movements Release Afflictive Emotions from Your Organs

Three proven exercise techniques have been combined—movement, breathing, and sounds—into what are called the Five Animal Forms. These movements and sounds send healing vibrations of Qi through the energetic system to rejuvenate the entire body through a combination of body and eye movements, abdominal breathing, and vibrating sounds that use specific placements of the tongue. This combination may help to prevent some signs of dementia, as the combination facilitates an essential flow of blood and oxygen to the brain. The internal movement of Qi promotes the flow of blood and oxygen, while the external movements can help to realign the posture and expand the chest, allowing the upper lung and lower abdominal areas to expand and contract naturally and help vital energy flow throughout the body.

In the Five Animal Forms exercises there are five animals: tiger, monkey, bear, bird, and deer. Their natural movements and sounds are mimicked in the movements of the exercises. In the Chinese medical tradition of Qigong, these animals represent five pairs of vital organs in the body. The movements and sounds of each animal stimulate organ energy in each pair, clearing them of blockages and allowing vital Qi to flow through newly opened channels.

Afflictive emotions can get trapped in each of the following organ pairs:

- anger disrupts liver and gallbladder energy

- joy (see page 18) clenches heart and small intestine energy

- worry blocks spleen and stomach energy

- grief stagnates lung and large intestine energy

- fear restricts kidney and bladder energy.[1]

The Five Animal Forms assist in releasing these negative emotions to bring about a healthy balance in organ energy. Although it might at first seem awkward to roar like a bear, sound therapy is a very ancient method of healing that can easily be integrated into Western practices for improved health—not to mention that the animal sounds are downright fun!

---

1   See Shen-Nong (2006) in Further Reading for more information.

**TABLE 7.1. FIVE ANIMAL CHART**

| ANIMAL | TIGER | MONKEY | BEAR | BIRD | DEER |
|---|---|---|---|---|---|
| **Characteristic** | Courageous | Smart | Humble | Compassionate | Perceptive |
| **Yin Organ** | Liver | Heart | Spleen | Lung | Kidney |
| **Yang Organ** | Gallbladder | Small intestine | Stomach | Large intestine | Bladder |
| **Sound** | GRR-R-R-R | HA-HA-HA | ROAR-R-R- | CAW-CAW | CLICK-CLICK |
| **Emotion Released** | Anger | Joy* | Worry | Grief | Fear |

* See page 18

Practicing these movements and sounds on a regular basis helps remove emotional blockages in organ energy. The sounds vibrate through the energy of the organs to release blockages that hold negative emotions. This makes it easier for energy, blood and oxygen to make their way around your body to provide natural healing and revitalized energy.

It takes about ten minutes to do the Five Animal Forms; fifteen minutes is even better.

For the purpose of this book, the Five Animal Forms are intended to be done while sitting comfortably in a chair. It is the safest way to model the helpful exercises for people with any type of memory loss, dizziness, imbalance, or frailty.

Grandchildren particularly like joining in and doing the sounds and movements, making for a multi-generational and healthy good time!

One example illustrates how everyone loves doing the animal sounds and movements. At the Memory Care Center one day, as the class broke out into roars, muffled roars could be heard in return from the people sitting in a lounge far down the hallway. By the end of the five exercises, the class size had doubled from the others coming down the hall to join in—a sort of call of the wild.

The Five Animal Form exercises on the next five pages are contributed by the Natural Healing Research Foundation as taught in their Senior Wellness Program with additional advanced practice for caregivers and others.

## BE THE TIGER

### Release anger from your liver with a "GRR...RR...RRR"

Anger gets trapped in the liver and gallbladder. When you make a deep-throated "GRR...RR...RRR" like a tiger, you release anger and feel a sense of calm.

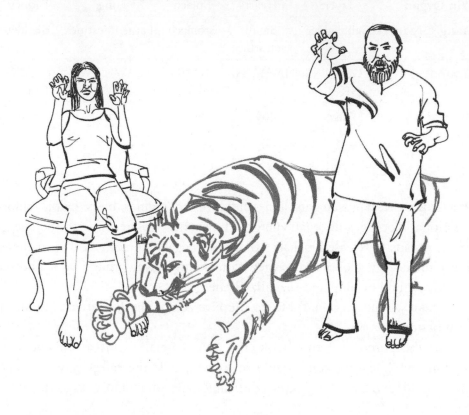

1.  Curl your fingers tightly into Tiger claws.

2.  Set your face with a look of Tiger intent.

3.  Raise your hands straight up in front of you as you take in a deep breath.

4.  Make a deep-throated "GRR...RR...RRR."

5.  Stretch one Tiger claw out in front of you and pull it back as you "GRR...RR...RRR."

6.  Then reach out with your other Tiger claw as you "GRR...RR...RRR."

7.  Do at least five sets of the Tiger movements and sounds as you imagine your liver and gallbladder rumbling.

**Advanced practice:**

1.  Lightly bite down on the sides of your tongue when "GRR...RR...RRRing."

2.  Look with piercing Tiger eyes when you do this animal sound.

3.  Open your "claws" widely when you stretch your arms out in front of you.

## BE THE MONKEY

### When your heart is robbed of joy, release the agitation with a "HA-HA-HA"

A deficiency or excess of joy traps agitation in the heart and small intestines, creating stress in the energy of those organs.

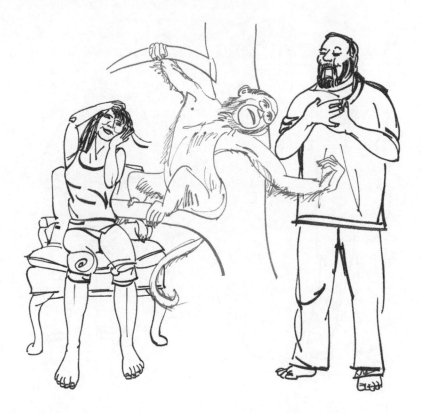

1. Rub your hands together to warm them up.

2. Place your warm hands over your heart and breathe in deeply.

3. Turn to one side and laugh out a "HA-HA-HA."

4. Then turn to the other side and laugh out a "HA-HA-HA."

5. Look forward, place your hands above your ears and hold your head.

6. Laugh out a "HA-HA-HA-HA-HA" as you rock back and forth, scratching your head.

7. Do at least five sets of the monkey movements and laughing sequence as you imagine your heart and small intestines lighting up with good energy.

### Advanced practice:

1. Press your tongue against the backs of your lower teeth when you "HA-HA-HA."

2. Blink with Monkey eyes each time you say "HA."

## BE THE BEAR

### Release worry from your spleen and stomach with a "ROAR...RR...RRR"

Worry gets trapped in the spleen and stomach. That tension is released when you "ROAR...RR...RRR" like a bear, making your worries go away.

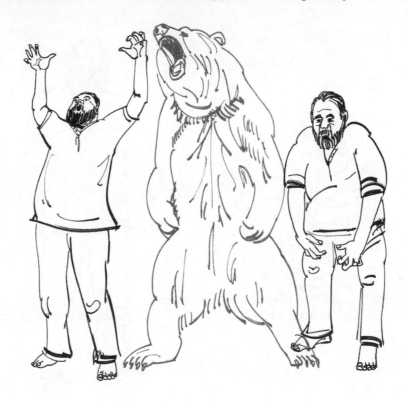

1. Rub your hands together to warm them up.

2. Cup your hands and stretch your fingers out slightly into heavy Bear paws.

3. Place your warm hands over your stomach and breathe in deeply.

4. Bow down and then raise your body up and bring your heavy Bear arms up over your head as you tilt backwards.

5. Force out a loud "ROAR...RR...RRR."

6. Do at least five of the Bear movements and sounds, "ROAR...RR...RRRing" louder and louder as you feel your stomach relax.

**Advanced practice:**

1. Place your tongue in the center of your mouth without letting it touch anything.

2. Keep your Bear eyelids half-closed and heavy.

3. Make the Bear movements without moving your eyes.

## BECOME THE BIRD

### Release grief from your lungs with a "CAW-CAW-CAW"

Grief gets trapped in the lungs and large intestines, which creates blockages. When you "CAW-CAW-CAW" like a bird, you release grief and tension.

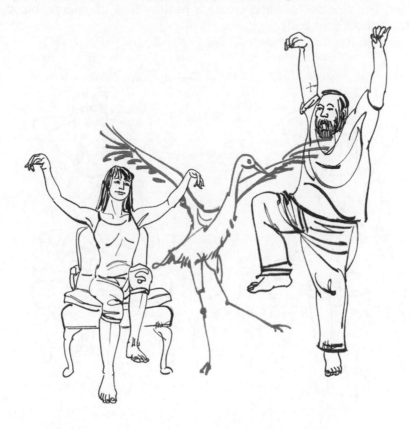

1. Spread your arms up and out like the wings of a crane.

2. Sing out a high-pitched "CAW" with every lift of your wings.

3. Lift one knee up toward your stomach at the same time as raising your arms.

4. Alternate the leg you pick up each time you "CAW."

5. Feel your lungs and large intestine expand with good energy as you feel like a bird looking down at the earth.

6. Do at least five sets of the bird movements and sounds to clear your lungs.

**Advanced practice:**

1. Push your tongue slightly out between your teeth as you "CAW."

2. After you finish "CAWing," roll your eyes around clockwise five times, and then counter clockwise five times.

## BECOME THE DEER

### Strengthen your kidney with a "CLICK-CLICK-CLICK"

Fear gets trapped in the energy of the kidney and bladder, which can cause blockages in the flow of energy to other organs. When you "CLICK-CLICK-CLICK" like a deer, you release fear and create a healthy flow of energy, blood and oxygen throughout your body.

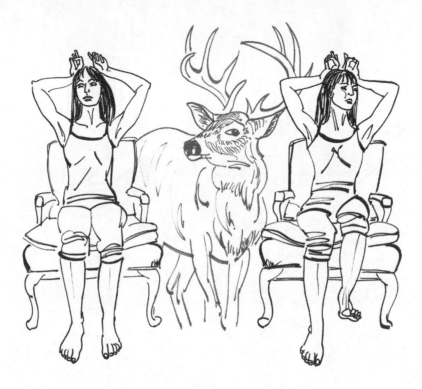

1.  Make Deer-like ears by pressing your thumbs and middle fingers together.

2.  Squeeze your fingers and thumbs together each time you say "CLICK."

3.  Alert like a deer in the forest, raise your "Deer ears" to the top of your head.

4.  Twist to one side and then the other, saying "CLICK-CLICK-CLICK" as you turn.

5.  Step quietly on the ball of one foot, and then the other, with each "CLICK."

6.  Do at least five Deer movements and sounds, and feel the muscle region around your kidneys warm with each twist of your waist.

**Advanced practice**

1.  Press the tip of your tongue into the roof of your mouth behind your front teeth each time you say "CLICK."

2.  When you finish the moves and sounds, look from left to right, right to left, at least five times without moving your head.

# 8

# Facial Massage Exercises to Wash Your Body with Energy

## Relax and Revitalize with a Facial "Energy" Massage

From the outside your face tells about the condition of your inside. New lines and wrinkles on your face can reveal signs of stress. That stress also affects your organ energy; you can't see the damage, but you can feel the tightness. The Facial Massage Exercises can stimulate organ energy to bring oxygen, blood, and energy to the skin, hair, and brain.

Most of your internal organs have representative points on your face and head, so when you relax or massage those points, the corresponding organs relax also. Just try it: breathe gently and let your face relax; let go of all the muscle tension in your face. Breathe out and then in…let relaxation come into your cheeks…your eyes…your forehead. Let your lips and jaw relax…your ears and top of your head, too. Now feel how your inner body has let go—it has relaxed at the same time, too!

The deep furrow that can appear between your eyebrows shows stress from anger in the liver and agitation in the heart. Your liver and heart have begun to release tension when your face relaxes. Relaxing the tightness from around your lips releases worry from the spleen and stomach, bringing calmness to your lips and those organs. When these facial exercises are practiced regularly, your face looks younger, your organ energy functions more smoothly, and, even more importantly, the relaxation response helps you think more clearly. Health and vitality radiate in a newly relaxed face, inner self, and mind. Simple and easy enough to practice often!

The face is dotted with reflexology, acupressure, and meridian points that can affect internal organ energy. Massaging these points on the face and head with warm hands can accomplish an energy exchange that may stimulate the good flow of energy, blood, and oxygen, not only in the face but throughout the entire body.

1. Combing the scalp activates energy flow in all of the meridians.

2. Circling the bone areas above and below the eyes affects Liver energy.

3. Massaging points along the nose can replenish Lung energy.

4. Manipulating the ears can improve Kidney energy.

5. Massaging the middle of the cheek supports Stomach energy.

6. The entire lip area stimulates Spleen energy.

7. Wiping off the chin connects to areas of the lower torso.

8. Stroking down the neck improves the flow of energy between the upper and lower body.

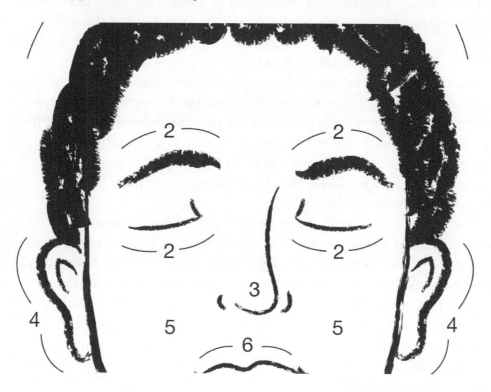

# 10 FACIAL EXERCISES

*Contributed by the Natural Healing Research Foundation*

According to Traditional Chinese Medicine, meridians are channels through which energy circulates in the body. They are also called "vitality pathways." The meridians connect different organs and systems of the body through a specific organization of networks. When energy circulates freely throughout these networks, it supports good blood circulation and allows the body to be well nourished so that it can function optimally.

As people age, the functions of facial sensory organs diminish, causing poorer eyesight, shorter and shallower breathing, weaker hearing, and a duller sense of smell and taste. This deterioration is due to aging and degeneration of internal organs. TCM theory describes how internal organ energy affects the sensory functions: liver energy affects the eyes and eyesight; kidney energy affects the ears and hearing, bones, teeth, and hair (thinning and loss as well as change in color to grey and white); lung energy affects the nose (duller sense of smell, shorter breaths, snoring, sleep apnea); and spleen energy affects the taste (duller sense of taste). The Facial Exercises are designed to address these physical conditions and can be beneficial when practiced regularly.

## 1. WASH YOUR FACE

1. Rub your hands together to gather warmth and energy.

2. Place your fingertips on your eyebrows so your hands cover your eyes and cheeks.

3. From this position, circle your hands UP and AROUND to make large circles that massage both sides of your face.

4. Repeat this circular massage nine times to wash your face with energy.

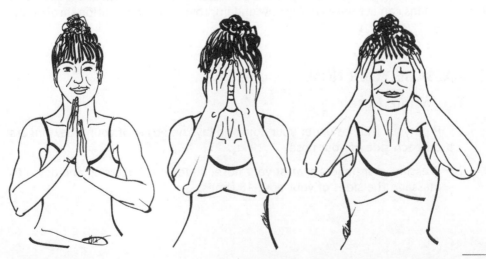

*Benefits:* As we age, the circulation of facial blood and energy decreases, which results in loss of skin firmness, lack of elasticity and luminosity, fine lines and wrinkles. According to TCM, there are many meridians that run through the face. When blockages occur, energy circulation is impaired. This energy deficiency decreases blood circulation to the organs. When you replenish energy to your face from your hands, it increases the circulation of energy and blood, which creates a cosmetic and nourishing effect to maintain a vibrant look.

## 2. COMB YOUR HAIR

1. Using your fingers like they are combs, place your fingertips along the top of your forehead and comb your hair from the top of your forehead to the base of your neck. Repeat this combing 18 times.

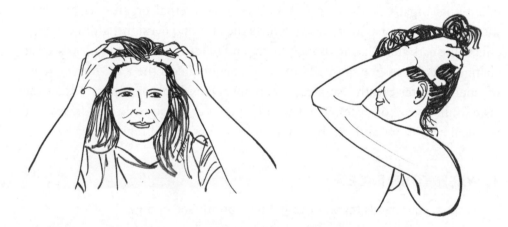

*Benefits:* All of the meridians gather in the head. When the fingers are used to comb through the hair, it stimulates the scalp and activates energy flow. This motion improves the circulation of energy and blood to the head, which is especially helpful for people with memory loss, forms of dementia, brain disorders, cardiovascular disease, kidney disease and diabetes. Using energy from the hands to stimulate the many reflex points on the head to clear blockages in the meridians can activate energy flow and improve blood circulation throughout the body.

## 3. MASSAGE YOUR NOSE

### A. The Whole Nose

1. Prop your thumbs under your chin and lay the edges of your index fingers on each side of your nose.

2. Pressing your fingers against your nose, slide your fingers up and down to massage the sides of your nose 18 times.

## B. Lower Nose Points

1. Place the tips of your index fingers in the crease of your nostrils on either side of your lower nose.

2. Make small circles with your fingertips, 9 times inward and 9 times outward.

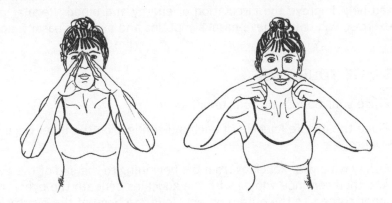

## C. Bridge of the Nose

1. Place the tips of your index fingers halfway up the sides of your nose. Press gently into the soft spots along the sides of the bridge.

2. Make small circles with your fingertips, 9 times inward and 9 times outward.

## D. Upper Nose Points

1. Place the tips of your index fingers at the top of your nose by the inner corners of your eyes.

2. Gently press on this area and make small circles, 9 times inward and then 9 times outward.

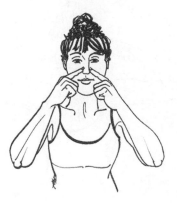
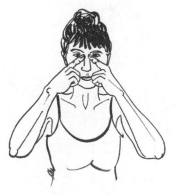

*Benefits:* The nose is the gateway to our respiratory system. Conditions such as nasal congestion, nasal allergies, sinus problems, snoring and sleep apnea affect the respiratory and cardiovascular functions. Due to poor respiration, the body can be deprived of sufficient oxygen, which may contribute to cardiovascular problems. There are many reflex points surrounding the nasal area. The upper nose points are located on the bladder meridian. The lower nose points are located on the large intestine meridian. Using the hands to stimulate these points can help improve the circulation of energy and blood. Regular practice of this exercise will help relieve nasal symptoms and improve nasal functions.

## 4. MASSAGE YOUR EYES

1. Place your thumbs on your temple.

2. Place the middle knuckle of each index finger on the inner edge of your eyebrows.

3. Firmly wipe your knuckles from the beginning to the end of the eyebrow. And then continue wiping with the knuckles beneath the eyes, from the inner corners to the outer corners along the bone of the eye sockets.

4. Repeat this massage 18 times.

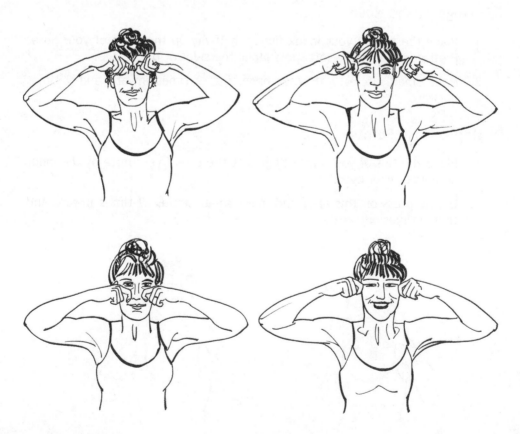

*Benefits:* Eye problems can be due to the degeneration of internal organs, which may contribute to the following: near and far sightedness, astigmatism, as well as common eye ailments such as cataracts, glaucoma, and macular degeneration. According to TCM, these conditions are attributed to blockages in the meridians of the gallbladder/liver, stomach/spleen, bladder/kidney and Governing Vessel. This energy deficiency will manifest physically as tender reflex points along these meridians. Using the energy from your hands to clear blockages and replenish energy in these meridians will help improve the condition of your eyes.

These eye massages wipe away fatigue and stress from your eyes and your liver.

## 5. MASSAGE YOUR CHEEKS

1. Make fists with your hands and point your thumb knuckles towards your face.

2. Place your thumb knuckles in the corners of your mouth and slide them up to a spot just under your cheekbones.

3. You'll know you are at the correct spot because it's a little tender. This is a stomach meridian point.

4. Circle your thumb knuckles on this point 9 times inward and 9 times outward.

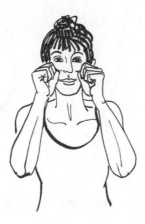

*Benefits:* As people age, they develop "bags" under their eyes and their sense of taste diminishes. This can be due to the weakening of the digestive system and deficient spleen energy. Using the energy from your hands to clear blockages and replenish energy to these meridians may help improve the digestive system. Also, regularly stimulating these two sensitive points may help to provide a youthful facial appearance.

## 6. MASSAGE YOUR EARS

### A. Pull Gently on Your Ears

Note: Keep your head straight with your eyes looking forward.

1. Reach your right hand over the top of your head and grasp the top of your left ear.

2. Scoop your left hand under your chin and grasp your right earlobe. Don't let go.

3. Simultaneously pull up and down 9 times on each ear. Let go.

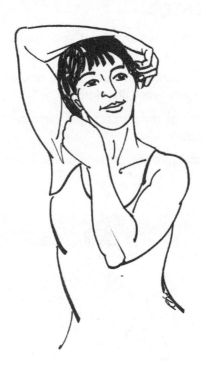

4. Reach your left arm over the top of your head and grasp the top of the right ear.

5. Scoop your right hand under your chin and grasp your left earlobe. Don't let go.

6. Simultaneously pull up and down nine times on each ear. Let go.

*Benefits*: According to TCM theory, the ear is the gateway to the kidneys. It also represents the entire body. Health issues such as ringing in the ears and hearing loss are common among middle age to older people, as their kidney energy becomes weaker. Surrounding the ear are the gallbladder/liver, and small intestine/heart meridians. When these meridians are blocked, they contribute to ringing in the ears and hearing loss. This exercise clears blockages, replenishes energy, and improves the circulation of energy and blood.

## B. Beat the Drum

1. Place your palms flat against your ears and hold the back of your head with your fingers.

2. Stretch your elbows out to the side and relax your shoulders as you press your palms against your ears.

3. Place your index fingers over your middle fingers.

4. Snap your index fingers against your head. It will sound loud like a drum inside your head.

5. Repeat the snapping 18 times.

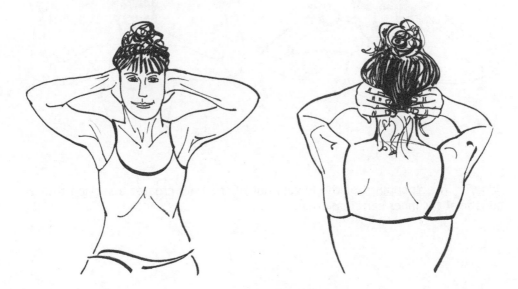

*Benefits*: Common complaints such as forgetfulness, brain fog, and memory loss, are due to insufficient oxygenation of the brain, which can accelerate the deterioration and death of brain cells. If left unchanged, it can lead to brain atrophy and serious brain disorders, such as dementia and Alzheimer's disease. From the TCM perspective, cardiovascular and kidney diseases are due to blockages in the Governing Vessel, bladder, gallbladder, and triple heater meridians. When these four meridians are blocked, energy becomes deficient. When you press your palms against your ears, it creates negative pressure that can stimulate the inner ear. Snapping your index fingers against your head creates a surge of energy within the head, and this vibration resonates with the energy of the brain. Further, this particular exercise replenishes energies, clears blockages, and improves inner ear circulation.

## C. "POP" the Cork

1.  Gently insert an index finger into each ear with your palms facing toward the floor.

2.  Twist your palms toward the front so that your fingers plug your ears.

3.  Quickly "POP" your fingers out of your ears.

4.  "POP" the finger-cork from your ears 9 times.

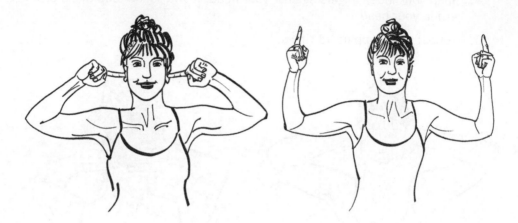

*Benefit*: The "popping" of the fingers out of the ears creates a suction that is beneficial for inner ear circulation.

## 7. MASSAGE KEY ENERGY POINTS

1. With your mouth closed, place the tip of your tongue behind your upper front teeth. This connects an energetic cycle between the Governing and Conception Vessels.

2. Place the tip of one index finger between your nose and upper lip.

3. Place the tip of the other index finger just below the center of your lower lip.

4. Simultaneously massage both points 9 times in clockwise circles and then 9 times in counterclockwise circles.

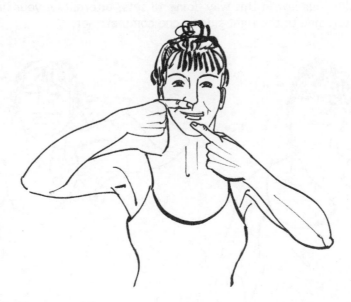

Note: The area where these two energy points are located is full of capillaries. Check with your doctor if you have swelling or infection around your mouth, as it can lead to sepsis.

*Benefits:* According to TCM, the first energy point above the lip is located on the Governing Vessel. Massaging this point can be used as a first-aid point in the emergency treatment of seizures, heat strokes and loss of consciousness. The second energy point, below the lip, is located on the Conception Vessel. The two points are similar to electrical switches in regulating the energy circuit in the body. These two points are important connecting points for the Governing and Conception Vessels, and are especially beneficial for the brain. Stimulation of these two energy points improves the circulation of energy and blood throughout the body. Those who experience memory loss from dementia and Alzheimer's disease have low kidney energy. Kidney energy controls the bone, teeth, bone marrow, and the brain.

## 8. WIPE YOUR CHIN

1.  Take your left hand and place it under your right ear so your hand rests along your jawbone from your ear to your chin.

2.  Pull your left hand along the jawbone completely across to the opposite ear, raising your elbow as high as you can.

3.  Take your right hand and place it under your left ear so your hand rests along your jawbone from your ear to your chin.

4.  Pull your hand along the jawbone completely across to the opposite ear, raising your elbow as high as you can.

5.  Stroke your jaw in this way doing 18 sets, alternating your hands from the left side to the right side as one complete set.

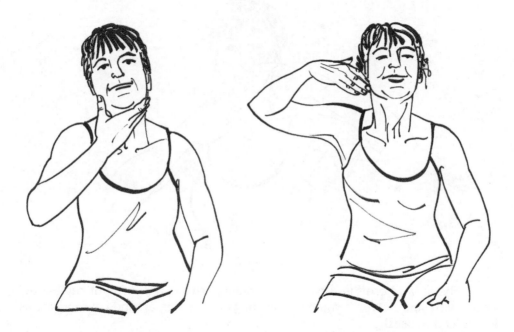

*Benefits:* According to TCM, the chin represents conditions of the torso and lower body. Several meridians flow through this area. In physiognomy (facial reading), the chin represents the latter part of one's life. A full chin, with rosy color and luminous skin, represents prosperity and longevity.

## 9. BRING ENERGY DOWN

1.  Tilt your head back and look toward the ceiling.

2.  Place your hands under your chin and then sweep one hand down your neck toward your lower abdominal area ending below your belly button.

3.  Now sweep the other hand down your neck to the lower abdominal area. At the same time, bring the first hand back under your chin.

4.  Alternate hands doing one sweep at a time.

5.  Repeat 12 sets of sweeps.

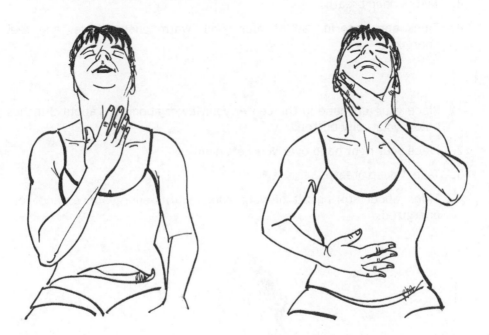

*Benefits:* The neck is where the throat, thyroid gland, trachea (windpipe), esophagus and major blood vessels are located. When you tilt your head and look up, this movement realigns the cervical vertebrae and stretches the neck muscles. As people age, swallowing may become difficult due to blockages in the throat. This exercise helps improve the circulation of energy and blood to this important area. The neck functions like a traffic hub that connects the head and the rest of the body and allows energy and blood to flow back and forth between the two.

## 10. CLOSING MEDITATION

Always do the following closing exercise after completing the Facial Exercises to store the energy you have gathered.

*Women:*

1. Place your right hand in the center of your lower abdomen, about 3 inches below your belly button.

2. Place your left hand over your right hand.

3. Take 3 deep breaths.

4. Think about storing all of your good, warm energy here, and feel energized.

*Men:*

1. Place your left hand in the center your lower abdomen, about 3 inches below your belly button.

2. Place your right hand over your left hand.

3. Take 3 deep breaths.

4. Think about storing all of your good, warm energy here, and feel energized.

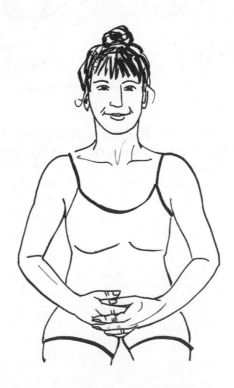

*Benefits:* Use your intent to direct your energy toward the lower dan tian (lower abdominal area, about 3 inches below belly button) in order to store the energy you have created in these exercises. According to Daoism, the lower dan tian is an energy reflexology center that promotes good health and longevity. The middle dan tian, located in the middle of the chest, controls the body and wisdom. The upper dan tian is located between the eyebrows and governs the brain and spirit.

Some people refer to Qigong as "Breath Exercise"

While the intention is to breathe comfortably, letting your breath come naturally, here are a few tips in case you need help.

**Abdominal breathing**

Begin with a long exhale to empty the lungs and collapse your tummy toward the spine. Then inhale slowly through the nose and draw your breath in, so that your entire abdominal area rises. As you continue to breathe in, air will fill your lungs from front to back and side to side until the breath reaches your collarbone. Don't strain. Slowly release the air from your lungs, and let your breathing develop into a comfortable rhythm of inhales and exhales.

# 9

# Twelve Sitting Exercises

*Meditation and Motion to Move
Energy Through Your Body*

If your energy is strong, no illness can befall you.

*The Yellow Emperor's Classic of Internal Medicine*, 300 BCE

Variations of the Twelve Sitting forms have been practiced for centuries as a form of medical Qigong meant to improve health through quieting the mind and body. This is important for being able to consistently channel energy through the lower abdominal area, known to the Chinese as the lower dantian, which supports longevity.

Each of the twelve exercises is based on the principle of easing tension in the body, which allows the parasympathetic response to help the body find the peace it needs to heal itself. The Twelve Sitting Exercises—Meditation and Movement—start with a form known as Baby-fists. This pose, with your thumbs tucked into the palms of your hands and then covered with your fingers, seals healing energy into your body.

The Twelve Sitting Exercises also help to stimulate the formation of saliva. With aging, our mouths begin to dry. Doing exercises that stimulate the production of saliva can be essential to our wellbeing by making swallowing easier, exciting our taste buds, aiding digestion and supporting immunity. Saliva is also excellent for the kidneys.

The simple movements of the Twelve Sitting Exercises massage internal organs to relieve ailments ranging from arthritis and asthma to dementia and allergies. These exercises are beneficial to anyone who is interested in living a naturally healthy life. And they are particularly helpful to anyone who may struggle with standing exercises or is experiencing any debilitating health issue. It is not uncommon to see people start out being able to do only sitting exercises; but when they experience improved health, some incorporate other forms of Qigong into their lifestyle. The Twelve Sitting Exercises are easy to do, and work to provide relief from painful symptoms, improve sleep, and calm nerves, all of which support clearer thinking. Allow yourself twenty minutes of quiet a few times a week to build healing energy.

When you first learn the Twelve Sitting Exercises, start by doing a few at a time with the intention of building up to complete all twelve exercises in one sitting. The descriptions are easy to follow, but the details can make them appear daunting. Always check with a doctor before starting a new exercise program.

## 12 SITTING EXERCISES
*Contributed by the Natural Healing Research Foundation*

## ONE: BABY-FISTS MEDITATION

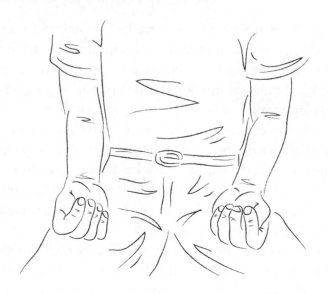

1. Sit comfortably in a straightbacked chair. The priority is to be comfortable.

2. Open your hands out in front of you, with your palms facing up.

3. Bend your thumbs towards the middle of each palm and fold your fingers over each thumb to make relaxed "Baby-fists."

4. Rest your "Baby-fists" on your lap with your closed fingers facing up. Breathe.

5. Place the tip of your tongue on the roof of your mouth behind your front teeth.

6. With your lips closed, let your mouth smile. It relaxes your face and opens your heart.

7. Breathe in and out comfortably throughout this meditation. If your breathing can come naturally from your abdomen, even better.

8. Meditate with happy thoughts, pleasant memories from the past. As you have these thoughts, relax your cheeks, relax your ears, relax your jaw, relax the top of your head. Let that relaxation ease into your shoulders and flow down your arms to your "Baby-fists." Feel it travel into your hips and down your legs to your feet. Breathe in and out with your happy thoughts as you let your eyelids close gently, and relax for the next few minutes or more.

9. Stretching to end "Baby-fists" Meditation:

   • Open your "Baby-fists" and clasp the fingers of both hands together.

   • Bring your hands up and behind your head with elbows out to the sides.

   • Breathe in and out nine times with your eyes closed.

*Benefits:* This exercise helps to calm the mind and eliminate distracting thoughts. Your intent to relax your body gradually moves energy down by directing it from your head to your feet. Positive thoughts may improve the circulation of energy and blood throughout the body to create a rejuvenating effect.

## TWO: BITING YOUR TEETH TO MAKE SALIVA

1. Make Baby-fists by touching your thumbs to the middle of the palms of your hands, palms facing up, and then closing your fingers over your thumbs.

2. Rest your Baby-fists comfortably on your lap, with your closed fingers facing up.

3. Gently close your lips together and relax your face and jaw.

4. Without opening your lips, open and close your teeth slowly 18 to 36 times, with your eyes softly closed.

5. Gather up the saliva that has collected in your mouth and swallow it down in one big gulp, feeling its warmth going into your stomach and beyond.

*Benefits:* "Biting your Teeth" can improve the energy flow in your jaw and mouth, which can be beneficial for temporo-mandibular joint problems. The "biting" stimulates the tooth bed and the formation of saliva, and is good for dry mouth problems. The additional saliva aids in the digestive process, too. This exercise also builds good energy for your liver and kidneys.

## THREE: BEAT THE DRUM

1. Place your palms flat against your ears and hold the back of your head with your fingers.

2. Stretch your elbows out to the side and relax your shoulders as you press your palms against your ears.

3. Place your index fingers over your middle fingers.

4. Snap your index fingers against your head. It will sound like a drum inside your head.

5. Repeat the snapping 18 times.

Benefits: Common complaints such as forgetfulness, brain fog, and memory loss, can be due to insufficient oxygenation of the brain, which may contribute to the deterioration and death of brain cells. If left unchanged, it can lead to brain atrophy and serious brain disorders, such as dementia and Alzheimer's disease. When you press your palms against your ears, it creates negative pressure that can stimulate the inner ear. Snapping your index fingers against your head creates a surge of energy within the head, and this vibration resonates with the energy of the brain. Further, this particular exercise replenishes energies, clears blockages, and improves inner ear circulation.

## FOUR: BENDING THE POST TO UNBLOCK YOUR ARM MERIDIANS

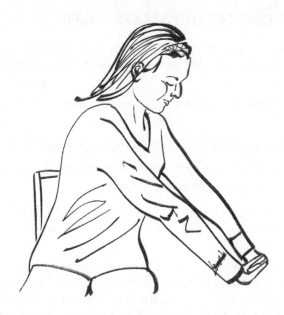

1. Inhaling, clasp your hands together in front of you so your palms face your heart.

2. Exhaling, twist from the waist to one side while turning your hands so your palms face away from you.

3.  Bend forward in that direction as you stretch your clasped hands out and slightly downward.

4.  Inhaling, pull your body back to the center and draw your hands back to the starting position.

5.  Repeat movements 1-4 in the same way to the other side.

6.  Do up to eight sets of these bends. Bending to one side and then to the other counts as one set.

To finish:

7.  Slide your clasped hands down the fronts of your legs, palms toward the floor, as you stretch downward.

8.  With your eyes looking downward, breathe in and breathe out completely for up to 9 breath cycles (one inhale-exhale is a cycle).

9.  Sit up, end with Baby-fists on your lap and take a few cleansing breaths.

*Benefits:* This exercise stretches the muscle regions of the three Yin meridians (lung, pericardium, and heart) and three Yang meridians (large intestine, triple warmer, and small intestine) of the arms. When you exhale and twist your waist, it moves abdominal energy through the arms and legs and is beneficial for clearing blockages. Bending forward from the waist, with proper breathing, changes the pressure within the abdominal cavity and creates a massage effect on the internal organs. This exercise may also help joint, digestive and circulatory problems.

# FIVE: GATHER SALIVA WITH YOUR TONGUE TO STRENGTHEN IMMUNITY

You will be circling your tongue around the fronts of your teeth in this exercise.

## Sitting with Baby-fists

1.  Make Baby-fists by touching your thumbs to the middle of your palms, and then closing your fingers over your thumbs.

2.  Rest your Baby-fists comfortably on your lap with your fingers facing upwards.

## The Tongue Movement

1.  Place your tongue completely over your upper front teeth and gums.

2.  Close your lips gently together.

3.  Circle your tongue completely around in one direction over the fronts of your upper and then lower teeth and gums making 9, 18, or 36 complete circles around your top and bottom teeth with your tongue.

4.  With your mouth closed, swish your saliva around, gather it up and swallow it in one big gulp.

5.  Inhale, and feel the saliva going to your lower abdominal area.

6.  Repeat the tongue circling in the opposite direction for the same number of times as the first set of circles. Gather your saliva and swallow it down in a gulp.

7.  Do a third set of tongue circles, going in the same direction as the first set of circles. Gather your saliva and swallow it down in a gulp.

8.  Once you feel comfortable doing this exercise, do it with your eyes closed.

*Benefits:* The tongue movement increases the secretion of saliva and helps strengthen the energy that supports digestion. By increasing saliva, you may also help your immune system, since two components of saliva have been shown to enhance immunity (Humphreys 2009). You are also strengthening the muscles involved in strong swallowing, which helps clear the central channel to promote energy flow down through the torso. This is important for being able to consistently build up and store energy in your lower energy center as a means to promote longevity.

## SIX: WARMING YOUR KIDNEYS FOR LONGEVITY

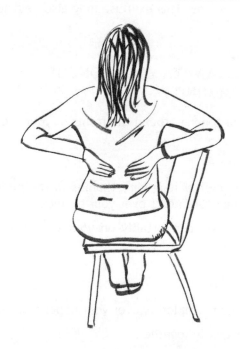

To do this exercise, first locate your kidney areas. They are on each side of your spine near the bottom of your rib cage, several inches above your waist. Place your hands over your kidney areas with your fingertips pointing toward your spine and your thumbs stretching toward the front. **If it is uncomfortable to put both hands on your back at the same time, do the following: Twist one side forward, place your hand on that kidney area and massage that side. Then twist the other side forward to massage that kidney area.**

1. Sit comfortably in a chair with your back as straight as possible.

2. Rub your hands together quickly to warm them up.

3. Place your warm hands over your kidney areas.

4. Rub up and down to massage your kidneys from 8 to 36 times.

5. Close your hands into Baby-fists and place them on your lap, fingers facing up.

6. Deeply exhale and inhale three times.

Once you are comfortable doing this exercise, gently close your eyes throughout all of the steps.

*Benefits:* The intent of visualizing your kidneys getting warm directs energy to that area. This may lessen ringing in the ears, calm the nerves, strengthen the bladder, and improve sleep. It also may improve the circulation of energy and blood to the area surrounding the kidneys.

## SEVEN: "COOKING THE PEARL" MEDITATION TO PROMOTE A LONG LIFE

1. Make Baby-fists by touching your thumbs to the middle of your palms, and closing your fingers over your thumbs.

2. Rest your Baby-fists comfortably on your lap, fingers facing up.

3. Place the tip of your tongue behind your top front teeth, lips relaxed in a smile, and keep your eyes lightly closed during the whole meditation.

4. Visualize the saliva you have swallowed being cooked into a smooth, warm pearl in your lower abdomen. Feel the warmth in your lower energy center as you inhale and exhale.

*Benefits:* This exercise will help promote a long, healthy life by relaxing your body and filling your lower energy center with vital energy. It may also improve the circulation of energy, blood, and oxygen that nourishes the body.

## EIGHT: A. CIRCLE YOUR ARMS

*Note:* If you have shoulder pain, do Exercise B on page 125 instead.

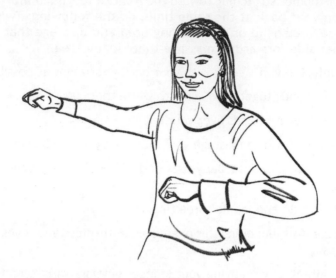

1. Make Baby-fists by touching your thumbs to the middle of your palms, and closing your fingers over your thumbs.

2. Rest your Baby-fists on your lap with your fingers facing up. Breathe.

3. Place the tip of your tongue on the roof of your mouth, behind your front teeth.

4. With your lips relaxed, let your mouth smile. It relaxes your face and opens your heart.

5. Raise one arm up, elbow bent so your Baby-fist is in front of your chest, fingers pointing down. *Accommodation:* If it is tiring to keep this arm up, rest your Baby-fist on your lap.

6. Raise the other Baby-fist out to your side, no higher than your shoulder, fingers toward the floor, with your index knuckle lower than your pinky knuckle.

7. Lean forward slightly in your chair.

8. Circle your arm up and backward, slowly drawing eight large circles with your elbow.

9. Inhale as you raise your arm. Exhale as you lower your arm.

10. Reverse, and circle the same arm up and forward, slowly drawing eight large circles with your elbow.

11. Inhale as you circle your arm up. Exhale as you circle your arm down.

12. Lower your Baby-fists to your lap, open your hands, and breathe deeply three times.

13. Reverse, and repeat movements 5 through 12 with your other arm.

14. To close: Rest your hands on your lap, palms up to release the stale energy and breathe deeply three times.

Once you are comfortable doing this exercise, gently close your eyes while circling your arms.

*Benefits:* This exercise clears energy blockages from the kidney, spleen, and liver meridians. It increases the flow of energy and blood to the chest and shoulder areas. The stretching of the shoulder, chest, and arm muscles helps to improve the circulation of energy and blood to the lungs and heart.

## EIGHT: B. SHOULDER ROLLS

1. Make Baby-fists by touching your thumbs to the middle of your palms and closing your fingers over your thumbs.

2. Rest your Baby-fists on your lap with your fingers facing up. Breathe.

3. Place the tip of your tongue on the roof of your mouth behind your front teeth.

4. With your lips relaxed, let your mouth smile. It relaxes your face and opens your heart.

5. Shrug your shoulders up and roll them backward to make eight complete circles.

6. Relax your shoulders and take one or two complete breaths.

7. Shrug your shoulders up and roll them forward to make eight complete circles.

8. Relax your shoulders and take one or two complete breaths.

## NINE: REACH FOR HAPPINESS TO BALANCE YOUR ENERGIES

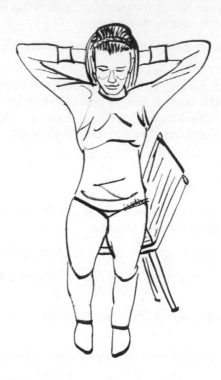

1.  Place the tip of your tongue on the roof of your mouth, behind your front teeth.

2.  With your lips relaxed, let your mouth smile. It relaxes your face and opens your heart.

3.  Sit comfortably up straight in a chair with your feet flat on the floor.

4.  Clasp your hands below your belly button with your palms facing up.

5.  Gaze at your hands as you raise them to face level.

6.  Rotate your hands away from you, inhale upwards and continue to raise your hands above your head, gazing at them as you raise them as high as you can.

7.  Lower your chin and exhale as you bring your clasped hands to the back of your head with your elbows out to the side.

8.  Tip your head backward to look up, and inhale as you raise your clasped hands above your head again, palms facing up.

9.  Lower your chin and exhale as you return your clasped hands to the back of your head. Repeat the sets of inhales and exhales six more times as you raise and lower your clasped hands.

10. Release your hands and return them to your lap in Baby-fists.

*Benefits:* This exercise balances the energies of the Triple Heater and the energies of all the internal organs. It lifts internal organs and can help to relieve tension in the shoulders and spine. It can be helpful for people who have foggy thinking, asthma, coughs, stiff neck, calcium deposits on the spine, diabetes, stomach bloating, and gas. It is also beneficial to the musculoskeletal and neural systems. Realigning the spine's cervical, thoracic, lumbar, and sacral areas regulates the circulation of energy and blood to the entire body.

## TEN: BEND YOUR BACK AND GRAB YOUR FEET TO MASSAGE YOUR ORGANS

1. Place the tip of your tongue on the roof of your mouth, behind your front teeth.

2. With your lips relaxed, let your mouth smile. It relaxes your face and opens your heart.

3. Sit near the edge of your chair and extend your legs straight in front of you. (If you feel at all unstable in your chair, use the accommodation below.)

4. *Accommodation:* When you first start to do this exercise, sit back in your chair with your feet flat on the floor and then spread your legs apart a little.

5. Rub your hands together to warm them up.

6. Place your warm hands on your knees.

7. Circle your hands around eight times one way, and then circle them around eight times the other way, to massage your knees.

8. Bend forward and slide your hands down your legs as far as you comfortably can.

9. While staying bent over, slowly inhale and exhale up to nine times from your abdomen.

10. Sit up and return your hands to Baby-fists on your lap and breathe deeply three times.

*Benefits:* This exercise massages the liver, kidney, and spleen as well as the stomach, gallbladder, and bladder. It especially supports the energies of the bladder, stomach, and the reproductive organs. It helps expand lung capacity and works to clear the energy blockages commonly associated with being overweight.

## ELEVEN: SWALLOWING SALIVA IN THIRDS FOR GOOD DIGESTION

1. Make Baby-fists by touching your thumbs to the middle of your palms, and closing your fingers over your thumbs.

2. Rest your Baby-fists on your lap, fingers facing up. Inhale deeply and exhale fully.

3.  With your lips relaxed, let your mouth smile. It relaxes your face and opens your heart.

4.  Close your eyes and think of sour foods—lemons...pickles...limes—and roll your tongue around in your mouth to gather a good amount of saliva.

5.  When you have a big ball of saliva, divide a third of it out and gulp that third of your saliva, holding the rest in your mouth.

6.  Breathe in deeply and exhale fully.

7.  Gulp the next third of saliva, holding the last third in your mouth.

8.  Breathe in deeply and exhale fully.

9.  Gulp the last third of saliva.

10. Clasp your hands below your belly button and breathe deeply three times as you think about the saliva going down into your energy center.

*Benefits:* This exercise helps strengthen the energy that supports your digestion. Also, two components of saliva have been shown to enhance immunity. Gulping strengthens the muscles involved in swallowing and helps clear the central channel and promote energy flow down through the torso to support longevity.

## TWELVE: LONGEVITY MEDITATION

**Women:**

1.  Place your right hand in the center of your lower abdomen, about 3 inches below your belly button.

2.  Place your left hand over your right hand.

3.  Roll your hands forward so your palms are facing up with your thumbs touching.

**Men:**

1.  Place your left hand in the center of your lower abdomen, about 3 inches below your belly button.

2.  Place your right hand over your left hand.

3.  Roll your hands forward so your palms are facing up with your thumbs touching.

### The Meditation

1.  Exhale fully, releasing tension from every part of your body.

2.  Inhale slowly, feeling your body fill up with new energy.

3.  Continue with slow, relaxed, and full abdominal breathing.

4.  Let your body fill with warming energy with every inhale, and let your body release tension and stale energy with every exhale.

5. Empty your mind of thinking and focus on your lower energy center.

6. Visualize storing the positive energy, which was created from the first 11 exercises, in the lower energy center.

7. Continue in this relaxed position for at least three minutes. Build up to at least ten minutes of meditation when you can.

8. Clasp your hands together and thank yourself for treating yourself well. Express your gratitude for others in your life.

9. Open your eyes with a renewed sense of calm and relaxed energy.

*Benefits:* The purpose of this exercise is to relax the body and calm the mind. The energy you are able to store in your lower energy center promotes longevity.

## TWELVE SITTING EXERCISES SIMPLE EASY

Following are condensed directions for the Twelve Sitting Exercises. The SIMPLE EASY descriptions are a quick reference guide to show how easy the Twelve Sitting Exercises are to do. The full descriptions already given provide details for enhancing the practice of each exercise.

### First Sitting Exercise SIMPLE EASY
**Baby-fists Meditation:** Sit comfortably with Baby-fists on your lap, your tongue resting behind your upper teeth and your lips in a relaxed smile. Think about happy memories, gently close your eyes and breathe comfortably for at least three minutes. Clasp your hands together and bring them behind your head. Breathe in and out nine times.

### Second Sitting Exercise SIMPLE EASY
**Biting Your Teeth to Make Saliva:** Sit with Baby-fists resting on your lap. Close your lips throughout the exercise. Bite down gently on your teeth and then slowly open your bite for 18 to 36 times with your eyes gently closed. At the end, gather up your saliva and quickly gulp it down.

### Third Sitting Exercise SIMPLE EASY
**Beat the Drum:** Press your palms over your ears and hold the back of your head with your fingers. Cross your index fingers over your middle fingers. Snap your index fingers to tap your head and make a drum sound. Drum 18 times.

### Fourth Sitting Exercise SIMPLE EASY
**Bending the Post to Unblock your Arm Meridians:** Clasp your hands together in front of your heart. Twist to one side as you turn your palms outward. Stretch them out and downward. Come back up to the starting position. Stretch in the same way to the other side. Do up to eight sets. To finish, bend forward and stretch your clasped hands toward the floor. Breathe up to nine complete times. Sit up and take a cleansing breath.

### Fifth Sitting Exercise SIMPLE EASY
**Gather Saliva with your Tongue to Strengthen Immunity:** Sit comfortably with Baby-fists on your lap, eyes closed. Circle your tongue around the front of your top and bottom teeth in one direction 9, 18, or 36 times, then gulp your saliva. Circle the same number of times the other way, and gulp your saliva. Circle your tongue the first way again the same number of times, and gulp. Breathe comfortably throughout.

### Sixth Sitting Exercise SIMPLE EASY
**Warming Your Kidneys for Longevity:** Warm your hands by rubbing them together. Place your hands over your kidney area. Close your eyes and massage this area up and down for up to 12 counts. Return Baby-fists to your lap, then deeply exhale and inhale three times.

### Seventh Sitting Exercise SIMPLE EASY
**"Cooking the Pearl" Meditation to Promote a Long Life:** Sit with Baby-fists resting on your lap, your tongue behind your upper teeth, and lips closed in a relaxed smile. Relax your face and then inhale and exhale deeply as you imagine a warm pearl forming in your lower abdomen. Continue this meditation, from a few minutes up to ten or more minutes.

### Eighth Sitting Exercise SIMPLE EASY
**Circle Your Arms:** Sit with Baby-fists on your lap. Raise one arm up, elbow bent, so your Baby Fist is in front of your chest, fingers pointing down. Raise the other Baby Fist out to your side, fingers toward the floor, with the index knuckle lower than the pinky knuckle. Draw eight large circles up and backwards with your elbow, inhaling as you go up and exhaling as you go down. Reverse direction and draw eight large circles up and forward, breathing the same way. Return your Baby-fists to your lap, open your hands and breathe deeply 3 times. Now repeat the exercise on the opposite side.

### Ninth Sitting Exercise SIMPLE EASY
**Reach for Happiness to Balance your Energy:** Clasp your hands below your belly button with your palms facing up. Raise your hands up toward your face. Turn your hands outward, inhale, and continue raising them above your head. Exhale as you lower your clasped hands behind your head, elbows back. Inhale as you raise your clasped hands up, and exhale as you lower your chin and return your hands behind your head. Do this exercise up to eight times. Return Baby-fists to your lap and breathe fully a few times.

### Tenth Sitting Exercise SIMPLE EASY
**Bend Forward and Grab your Feet to Massage your Organs:** Stretch your legs out. (Or, sit back in a chair with your feet flat on the floor and your legs spread slightly.) Warm your hands up and place them on your knees. Massage in circles one way eight times, then circle the other way eight times. Slide your hands down your legs. Take up to nine deep, slow, complete breaths. Sit up, return Baby-fists to your lap, and breathe deeply three times.

**Eleventh Sitting Exercise SIMPLE EASY**
**Swallowing Saliva in Thirds for Good Digestion:** Sit with Baby-fists resting on your lap. Relax your closed lips and smile. Roll your tongue around and think of sour foods to collect saliva in your mouth. Quickly gulp the saliva, one third at a time, taking one deep breath between each gulp. Return Baby-fists to your lap and take three deep breaths.

**Twelfth Sitting Exercise SIMPLE EASY**
**Longevity Meditation:** Sit comfortably with one hand resting over the other on your lap (men left over right; women right over left). Take full, deep and relaxed inhales and exhales and focus on the lower energy center. Breathe in this meditative pose for at least three minutes, building up to ten minutes. At the end, clasp your hands together and thank yourself and others for the beauty in life.

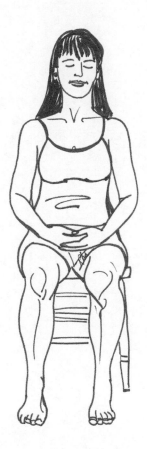

*For those of you who take care of your parents, you deserve the highest praise and thanks.*
Colorado Ombudsman

# PART III

Foods to Awaken
## NATURAL HEALING

# 10

# Introduction to the Chinese Understanding of Nutrition

Pick up any jar or container of food in a grocery store and you will see labels that give nutritional information based on recommended amounts, which include the following: calories, fats (saturated and trans), cholesterol, sodium, dietary fiber, sugars, and more. Practitioners of Traditional Chinese Medicine (TCM) have a different take on the adage, "You are what you eat." Rather than focusing on the amounts of things in foods, they seek out the essence—which foods address a person's specific needs during any given season, or day.

In Chinese tradition, foods are often considered medicine, and dietary considerations are based upon the need to balance an individual's yin and yang energies. For instance, a person experiencing a decline in kidney functioning can benefit from a food like Black Fungus that can bolster kidney energy, as well as the cardiovascular system. The goal is to balance yin with yang energy.

---

*It is important to know about the energies of food because different energies act upon the human body in different ways and affect our state of health. If a person suffers from cold rheumatism and the pain is particularly severe on a cold winter day, eating foods with a warm or hot energy shall relieve the pain considerably. Or if a person suffers from skin eruptions that worsen when exposed to heat, it is beneficial to eat foods with a cold or cool energy to relieve the symptoms.*

Yi (2006)

---

In Part I it was noted that the organs are associated with specific properties, including color, season, emotion and element; to these, taste can be added. TCM believes that the flavor of foods will facilitate the movement of energy to their matching organs:

## TABLE 10.1 ORGANS AND THEIR ASSOCIATED TASTES

| ORGANS | EMOTION | SEASON | COLOR | TASTE |
|---|---|---|---|---|
| Liver Gallbladder | Anger | Spring | Green | **Sour** |
| Heart Small Intestine | Joy (see page 18) | Summer | Red | **Bitter** |
| Spleen Stomach | Worry | Late summer | Yellow | **Sweet** |
| Lung Large Intestine | Grief | Autumn | White | **Pungent** |
| Kidney Bladder | Fear | Winter | Dark blue; black | **Salty** |

From TCM's perspective, a complete diet needs to include all five food tastes to help energy flow and nourish the organ associated with each taste.

- sour (cranberries, lemons, vinegar) promotes liver energy

- bitter (kale, artichoke, celery) balances heart energy

- sweet (quinoa, mangos, beef) strengthens spleen energy

- pungent (onions, ginger, bell peppers) feeds lung energy

- salty (black salt, seaweed, duck) sustains the kidney

However, some flavors might be augmented or diminished, depending on a person's individual needs, or even the time of year: during the yin months of winter, foods like red meat that generate heat might be preferable; while yin foods that are cooling, such as fish and vegetables, would be eaten during the summer months to balance out excessive yang.

Just as flavors confer energy benefits to specific organs, the colors of foods are also important, which might be hard for the Western mind to, well, swallow. Nevertheless, TCM believes that when you match the color of a food with the organ it represents, the essence of the food has a property that addresses the specific energy needs of that organ. The five yin organs dealt with in this book have corresponding food colors that are linked in this way:

- red foods (pomegranates, tomatoes, cherries) benefits heart energy

- yellow foods (turmeric, cantaloupe, sweet potato) protect spleen energy

- white foods (onions, garlic, pears) help clear congested lung energy

- dark foods (brown rice, walnuts, black mushroom) bolster kidney energy

- green vegetables (kale, spinach, broccoli rabe) promote liver energy.

Of course, a particular food can confer energy benefits to more organs than just the organ pair with which its color is associated according to the Five Element Theory. For example, foods rich in antioxidants come in all flavors and colors. But if one follows the suggestions in this book, the proof comes from the relief those foods bring from pain and discomfort.

For people with dementia, it is suggested to eat foods that address the root cause: low kidney energy. As we saw in Chapter 1, low kidney energy affects the bones and bone marrow. When red blood cell production from the bone marrow is diminished, the brain doesn't receive the oxygen it needs. Therefore, Qigong exercises and healing foods improve kidney energy and aid in the production of red blood cells in the bone marrow. Natural healing suggests foods that are high in protein, natural fiber, and vitamins; and it advises not to eat hydrogenated oils, processed fats, refined sugars, artificial sweeteners, and added refined salt or table salt. The best way to get salt essence for kidney function is naturally through foods like sea vegetables, celery, eggs, and saltwater fish or by adding a clamshell to soup. Sodium chloride is the major substance for maintaining the osmotic pressure of the human body. When the body lacks available sodium, symptoms such as fatigue, dizziness, vomiting, and abdominal pain might appear, which are signs of low salt syndrome. As Renneboog, Musch, and Vandemergel (2006) have confirmed, chronic salt syndrome (not enough salt in the body) is associated with falls, unsteadiness, and attention deficits. It is very important to check with your doctor about the appropriate levels of salt for your diet. Too much or too little can affect your health. If you must add a pinch of salt, make it unrefined sea salt.

For people who have begun to show degenerative signs of dementia, the NHRF program suggests foods to add to your diet that include roasted nuts and seeds like ground sesame seeds, gingko leaves, seeds and Chinese almonds (but not too many), walnuts and walnut oil, and lecithin-rich foods (see page 138) because they help blood circulation and nerve cell restoration. Avoid fried foods and foods with preservatives that over-excite brain cells. Lower vitamin D levels are linked to a higher risk of cognitive impairment, so it is good to enjoy the outdoor sun, as well as eating eggs. Drink green or herbal tea, exercise, and know that by following these recommendations, you are taking real steps toward wellbeing for yourself or loved ones that can enhance vitality. Make one or two changes at a time and the difference you feel will help you do more. Learn to listen to your body and it will take care of you.

Listening to your mind can lead you down a path of excuses; but when you listen to how food makes your body feel, you are on the road to wellbeing.

# Some Recommended Healing Foods

## 1. Foods for the Brain

When preparing a menu with the health of your brain in mind, the order of importance for what to include is:

- Seeds and nuts of all kinds—walnuts, hazelnuts, pecans, chia seed (soak first), flax seed, pistachio nuts, and almonds.

- Black fungus and all other mushrooms.

- Ocean vegetables, seaweeds (soak first), kelp, dulse, spirulina, algae—dried and powered forms are a good source.

- Vegetables, dark vegetables like black beans, spinach, chives, beets—whole and juiced.

- Unrefined oils such as sesame oil, coconut oil, extra virgin olive, grape seed oil, fish oils and avocados.

- In addition, add small portions of deep cold water fish: salmon, black cod and Chilean sea bass and search out foods that are rich in vitamin A, B2, B12, C, D, and E.

## 2. Foods to Improve Kidney Energy

- Toasted seeds (pine nuts, black sesame seeds), toasted almonds, roasted nuts and their oils, such as macadamia, walnuts, and hazelnuts—all of which may also help nerve cell regeneration (Windblad 2010), brown rice, black and long grain rice, barley, black mushrooms, sea cucumbers, goji berries, celery, lily flower, eggplant (aubergine), black beans. It is interesting to note that many of these foods that help the kidneys are predominantly dark blue or black.

### 3. Foods with Lecithin Benefit the Nerves and Speed Nerve Cell Recovery

- Seeds (need to be chewed), garbanzo beans (chickpeas), mushrooms, avocado, cabbage, cauliflower, broccoli, Brussels sprouts, kidney beans and black beans, Atlantic cod, salmon, egg yolk, dark chocolate.

### 4. Herbs and Spices with Anti-Inflammatory Properties

- Turmeric, which contains a form of curcumin, ginger, licorice, basil, rosemary, garlic, cayenne, cinnamon, and parsley for kidney ailments are highly recommended for their anti- inflammatory properties.

### A Few Tips About the Suggested Foods

- Bake all nuts and seeds in the oven for a few minutes, or lightly sauté them in a wok with no oil or water added.

- Use fresh mushrooms when possible and sauté in light oil so you don't eat them raw.

- Quickly sauté fresh greens and mushrooms in very light oil to make digesting them easier.

- Avoid using ice in drinks and eating cold foods. Warm foods, in essence and temperature, keep your stomach strong to make digestion smooth.

- Enjoy oils in moderation choosing unrefined oils whenever possible and light high-temperature oils for heated cooking. Include unrefined coconut oil in cooking and smoothies whenever you can. Other oils to keep on hand: walnut, sesame, cold pressed olive oil and grapeseed oil. Learn about cooking oils—they are an asset to your digestive and nervous systems.

In the remaining pages of this section, a selection of recipes is provided for family members and caregivers to prepare for the folks in their care. These recipes draw from many of the foods that have already been discussed. Experiment with adding your own ideas to the recipes. Your intuition will be your guide once you start to become familiar with foods that feed your organ energy. You will start to desire healthful foods more and more as you learn what to prepare for the one in your care. The foods listed are some of the more important foods to get started with. As you can see in the chart, not all foods match exactly the taste and color of the organ pairs, but remember, each food does support the functioning and interactions of the listed organs.

TABLE 10.2. THE ORGANS AND HEALING FOODS

| Kidney Bladder | Liver Gallbladder | Heart Small Intestine | Spleen Stomach | Lung Large Intestine |
|---|---|---|---|---|
| Black/dark blue | Green | Red | Yellow/orange | White |
| Salty | Sour | Bitter | Sweet | Pungent |
| Abalone | Bee pollen | Toasted almonds | Carrot | Cauliflower |
| Black beans | Broccoli rabe (Rapini) | Bitter melon | Chinese barley | Celery |
| Black sesame | Chicory | Broccoli rabe (Rapini) | Cinnamon | Chilli pepper |
| Cinnamon | Dandelion greens | Cinnamon | Corn | Garlic |
| Coarse salts | Eggplant (Aubergine) | Ginger | Dates | Honey |
| Deep sea fish | Endive | Ginko | Ginger | Leeks |
| Mushrooms | Fennel | Plum tomatoes | Lotus seed | Mushrooms |
| Mussels | Garlic | Red apples | Mango | Pears |
| Pine nuts | Lemon | Red beets | Pumpkin | Radish |
| Shellfish | Papaya | Red grapes | Shitake mushrooms | Scallions (Spring onions) |
| Walnuts | Scallions (Spring onions) | Sour cherries | Sweet potato | Turnips |
| Whole grains | Vinegar | Watermelon | Taro root | Water chestnuts |

# List of Some Healing Foods

*True healthcare begins in your kitchen.*

Anonymous

Make a copy of the following food list to carry with you to check which healing foods to add to your basket. As you shop you may be drawn to what you need. After eating according to the Five Elements, you may develop an intuition about the foods your energy needs to stay healthy.

- **Almonds** improve lung function.
- **Balsamic vinegar** strengthens the liver and spleen and improves sleep.
- **Cauliflower** increases kidney energy and strengthens lung function.
- **Celery** promotes calm sleep and reduces inflammation.
- **Chives** strengthen kidney energy and warm cold feet.
- **Cinnamon** reduces inflammation and helps blood sugar levels.
- **Eggplant (aubergine)** lowers cholesterol and clears large intestine.
- **Ginger** relieves digestive problems and improves circulation.
- **Goji berries** strengthen kidney energy and help reduce blood sugar.
- **Green tea** clears the mind and relaxes the liver.
- **Kelp** helps clear retained body fluids and adds iodine.
- **Kiwi fruit** improves liver function and strengthens the stomach.
- **Mushrooms** (fresh and lightly sautéed) support ALL organ systems.
- **Onions** help clear phlegm from the lungs and spleen.
- **Pears**, cooked or raw, are good to keep your digestive system active.
- **Plum tomatoes** are a healing food for heart, stomach, and liver function.
- **Red apples** improve metabolism and function of lung and intestines
- **Red grapes** invigorate Qi and enrich the blood and spleen.
- **Sesame seeds** (black) nourish the liver, eyes, brain and hair.
- **Scallops** strengthen the kidney and reduce frequent urination.
- **Strawberries** help to digest fat, improve sleep and circulation.
- **Sweet potato** helps digestion and bowel movements.
- **Walnuts** are powerful; they improve memory and kidney function.
- **Watermelon**, puree and drink to protect the heart and bladder.

*One must research every idea carefully, and not jump*
*to conclusion because other people say so.*

T'ao Hung-Ching, Chinese Herbalist, 452–536 CE

It has long been believed that food is the best medicine: "Let food by thy medicine, and thy medicine be food," advised Hippocrates, 300s BCE; China's Sun Si Miao, 500s CE, taught, "the doctor first tries to treat the illness with food"; and, in early 1900s America, Thomas Edison observed, "The doctor of the future will give no medicine, but will interest his patients in the care of the human frame, in diet as the cause and prevention of disease." An ancient Egyptian proverb sums it up best: "One quarter of what you eat keeps you alive. The other three quarters keeps your doctor alive."

From the earliest times into the present, the tradition of Chinese medicine has carried the principles of the Five Element Theory that include an interrelationship between the organs of the body and foods. When following some suggestions from reliable sources about the natural healing properties of foods, the results will inform your body. But, facing the challenge of changing some habits can seem daunting. And, listening to new ideas and suggestions can lead to confusion. Salt is a good example of this.

As you make nutritional changes, many more questions will come up. The best suggestion is to try new ideas slowly so you can see how the changes affect you. Try to keep your worries down, or work on releasing them, because digesting harmful emotions can be as harmful as digesting unhealthy food. Shop for food wisely and turn your pantry into a "Farmacy."

Always check with your primary care physician first, and ask questions about the health concerns you have. It is important to know if you have high blood pressure, diabetes, allergies, or other health concerns, so you and your doctor can make the best decisions for your wellbeing. It's your health, and learning more about how to be naturally healthy is worth the effort. A blending of approaches from both the East and the West may be the answer.

# 11

# Recipes for Rejuvenating Health

*Meals hold the energy—energy from both the food and the cook.*

*Preparing and cooking foods are essential practices of Qigong.*

*Ancient Chinese Wisdom, as told by Ruby, Chinese cook extraordinaire*

## Morning Juice

The body is a small universe, and, like the big universe of the earth, it is composed of more than 70 percent water. When the water of either universe becomes toxic, everything in the system eventually becomes weakened and sick. In the body the kidneys are responsible for cleansing the bodily fluids, and the large intestines eliminate solid body wastes. The NHRF's Morning Juice helps to clean the body by utilizing ingredients that strengthen the body's natural detoxification function. It is a simple, delicious, and profoundly nutritious drink that can help with daily bowel movements. The large intestine has been called a 'second brain' so it's smart to keep it moving.

Goji berries, also known as wolfberries, are an important ingredient in the Morning Juice and other recipes. They are very high in anti-oxidants and vitamins. The legendary Li Qing Yuen, of China, is said to have eaten goji berries in a soup every day, thus adding to the berry's popularity. Even at 130 years old he is said to have had keen sight, strong legs, and took vigorous walks every day. Often it is thought that when something is so good, more is better, but eat no more than half a cup of goji berries a day. It is suggested to look for the best source of the berries to ensure purity.

Check with your doctor if you have swollen ankles or other signs of fluid retention, or if you are taking blood thinners or drugs for diabetes or hypertension before adding new foods to your diet. If you are not certain that you should be eating goji berries, check with your doctor or an experienced TCM practitioner.

## The NHRF Morning Juice

It is best to drink the Morning Juice first thing every morning on an empty stomach. This helps the ingredients stimulate the digestive system. Often people have elaborate routines to prepare themselves for the day. Usually they shower, take care of their faces and brush their teeth, only focusing on their outer appearance. The Morning Juice helps to clean the internal body and adjust the pH levels to allow energy to be stronger for the whole day.

## Ingredients

- 12–15 goji berries to work as a blood and longevity tonic

- 1–2 teaspoons (5–10 ml) toasted walnut oil to benefit bones and brain function and aid in bowel movements; high in omega 3 fatty acids, vitamins, trace minerals and protein

- 1 tablespoon (15 ml) honey to benefit the digestive system

- ½ lemon, juiced, to support the liver and benefit the stomach

- 12 fl. oz. (360 ml) boiling water.

## To Make:

1. Rinse the goji berries very well and place them in the bottom of a 12 oz. (360ml) cup.

2. Pour enough boiling water into the cup to cover the goji berries and let them sit for 10 minutes. (You can keep soaked berries in a covered container in the fridge.)

3. Add the walnut oil, honey, lemon juice, and fill the remainder of the cup with warm water.

4. For increased benefits you may want to add a few pieces of thinly sliced Buddha's hand fruit or lemon to eat along with the goji berries to support the liver/gallbladder and stomach/spleen organ pairs.

Sit quietly to start the day, sip the juice and slowly chew the goji berries.

The NHRF considers that Morning Juice is a way to detoxify the body by balancing your pH levels, increasing blood circulation, stimulating the digestive system, and cleaning out old body fluids through the kidney and bladder pair. All of these improve your body's natural metabolism.

## NHRF Brain Mix: An Afternoon Snack for Kidney Energy

An afternoon snack should be for the purpose of strengthening kidney energy. The bladder and kidney hours of the day are from 3:00 to 5:00 p.m. and 5:00 to 7:00 p.m., respectively—a good time of the day for increasing kidney energy.

### Ingredients

- 1 cup (60 g) dried goji berries
- 1 cup (170 g) almonds
- 1 cup (120 g) walnuts
- 1/2 cup (60 g) black sesame seeds
- 1/2–3/4 cup (4–6 fl. oz) honey.

### To Make:

1. Heat oven to 250°F (120°C) and turn oven off.

2. Rinse goji berries and blanch them in boiling water. Drain well, roughly chop and spread wet goji on a cookie sheet. Place in warmed oven for 10 minutes or until goji are dried thoroughly to prevent spoilage.

3. After the goji berries have dried, turn the oven back on to 400°F (200°C)

4. Bake the sesame seeds at 400°F (200°C) until lightly toasted, and then grind in automatic grinder. Set aside.

5. Finely chop the almonds and walnuts and bake at 400°F (200°C) until lightly toasted.

6. In a small bowl, mix the honey with the dry ingredients.

7. Refrigerate in a covered bowl and then enjoy 1–3 tablespoons at a time.

8. Once cooled, the mixture can be rolled into balls and wrapped in plastic wrap for easy traveling to enjoy on the road or in the office.

This recipe can be doubled or tripled to have more on hand.

When choosing an afternoon snack, make it something with nuts, seeds, celery, blueberries, and foods that feed the kidney. It will feed the brain, too.


## Benefits of Ingredients in Brain Mix

- **Almonds** must be baked at 400°F (200°C) degrees until lightly toasted. You can do this yourself or purchase unsalted roasted almonds at the store. They improve digestion, increase blood circulation, have anti-cancer properties; they are also good for the lungs to ward off coughs, congestion, asthma, wheezing, and bronchitis. One serving contains nine per cent of the daily-recommended amount of calcium.

- **Walnuts**, baked at 400°F (200°C) until lightly roasted, nourish Kidney energy and essence, and also help cardiovascular health, the brain and cognitive functioning. They contain good amounts of alpha-Linolenic acid and Omega-3 fatty oils.

- **Black sesame seeds**, baked at 400°F (200°C) until lightly toasted to nourish kidney essence, strengthen hair and bones, and to promote longevity. Chew well or finely grind to prevent diverticulitis. Watch when baking, they toast quickly. Abundant in calcium and zinc.

- **Goji berries** have strong antioxidant properties and strengthen the liver, blood and eyes. They are especially good to tone the blood. An excellent fruit for longevity. Limit amount eaten to 1/2 cup per day.

- **Pine nuts** are loaded with potassium. Take care when baking, they toast very quickly.

Make it a little easier to have nourishing nuts and seeds on hand at all times:

- **Nuts and seeds** are the number one ingredient for nourishing your health, so spend a morning making batches ahead to add to salads, cereals, and other dishes or to put together a quick Brain Mix. Prepare large portions of the nuts and seeds as described, and then place them in airtight containers and pop them into the freezer. Glass containers are best because nuts easily absorb odors of other foods. Nuts can be kept from 18 to 24 months in the freezer; and the easy part is, they can be immediately put into a recipe straight from the freezer.

When baking seeds and nuts, just use your nose instead of watching the oven. As soon as you smell the delightful aroma of the seeds or nuts you'll know they are ready.

## Chinese Barley With Orange Marmalade

Chinese pearl barley, or coix seed (smaller and more nutritious than regular barley) has been proven to contain anti-cancer and anti-obesity properties (TCM World Foundation 2014). It is also very beneficial for digestion (stomach/spleen) and skin (lung/large intestine) . Barley takes time to prepare—boil up a batch ahead of time and store in refrigerator for later use.

## *Ingredients*

- 1 cup (250 ml) of Chinese pearl barley, rinsed well before cooking

- Five times the amount of water per amount of barley

- 1 apple, finely chopped*

- 4 heaped tablespoons (60–70 ml) of orange marmalade*

- ½ cup (125 ml) mayonnaise to taste*

- ½–¾ cup (70–100 g) toasted pine nuts*

- 1 scallion (spring onion), finely chopped.*

* Adjust amounts of ingredients to taste.

## *To Make:*

1. Cook the Chinese barley for 45 minutes to one hour. Drain off any remaining liquid and allow the barley to cool.

2. Bake the pine nuts at 400°F (200°C) until lightly browned.

3. Mix all the ingredients together: barley, apple, pine nuts, scallion (spring onions), marmalade, and mayonnaise.

4. Optional: Garnish with thin slices of orange.

For variety, add one or more of the following ingredients: dried sour cherries, roughly chopped, dried cranberries, roughly chopped, goji berries, well rinsed, soaked in boiling water and roughly chopped. You can halve, double, or triple the recipe, depending on how much you want. After trying it once, you'll probably want a lot more! It's even yummy for breakfast.

For more recipes like this, go to: www.tcmworld.org/dragonsway/the-dragons-way-recipes-for-self-healing.

## Cauliflower and Leek Soup

This is a warm and comforting soup to support the lungs and increase kidney energy. An excellent source of vitamin K, it acts as a direct regulator of inflammatory response. Leeks add important protection for blood vessels.

### Ingredients

- 1 head of cauliflower

- 3 leeks

- 5 mushrooms—assorted, small to medium-sized

- ½–¾ teaspoon (3–4 ml) turmeric

- ¼ teaspoon (1.5 ml) white pepper (freshly ground if available)

- 3 tablespoons (50 ml) grapeseed oil or other high-heat oil

- 1 cup of three coarsely chopped vegetables like Brussels sprouts, carrots, celery

- ½ cup shredded purple cabbage.

### To Make:

1. Remove any green leaves and the hard core of the cauliflower.

2. Coarsely chop the cauliflower florets, rinse, and put in a saucepan.

3. Cover with water and boil until tender.

4. Coarsely chop the mushrooms and set aside.

5. Remove green tops of the leeks and finely slice the white stalks, and set aside.

6. Heat grapeseed oil and pepper in a wok or medium frying pan.

7. Lightly sauté mushrooms and leeks in grapeseed oil until tender but not brown.

8. Drain the cauliflower over large pot; reserve the water.

9. Place all ingredients in a blender with 1–1½ cups (350 ml) of the reserved hot cauliflower water. Purée, adding more water as needed.

10. Sauté the chopped vegetable mixture in grape seed oil until sweated.

11. Add all ingredients to the saucepan, stir in the turmeric and simmer for 20 minutes.

12. Serve with a pinch of shredded purple cabbage on top. A few finely chopped pistachios make an added treat on top, too.

## Warm Greens and Spicy Pine Nut Sensation

A distinctive dish to add to fish or enjoy alone. It offers excellent support for liver and gallbladder energy. The multitude of ingredients provides a healthy side dish for all of your organ pairs.

*Ingredients:*

- ½ pound (225 g) broccoli rabe (rapini)
- ¼ pound (113 g) chicory or endive
- ¼ pound (113 g) dandelion greens
- 3 tablespoons (45 ml) coconut oil
- 3 large cloves garlic, minced
- 1 teaspoon (5 ml) fresh ginger, minced
- ½–¾ cup (40–60 g) coarsely chopped fresh mushrooms
- 3 tablespoons (45 ml) toasted pine nuts
- ½ teaspoon (2.5 ml) cinnamon

## *To Make:*

1. Clean all the greens and chop into 2–4-inch (5–10 cm) pieces.

2. Bring a pot of water to the boil.

3. Add broccoli to boiling water and cook for 2 minutes.

4. Add remaining greens and cook for another minute or less.

5. Drain greens completely and set aside.

6. Lightly toast pine nuts, black sesame seeds, and cinnamon in a small frying pan and set aside.

7. Heat a wok or shallow frying pan and add oil to coat the pan.

8. Add cayenne pepper and lightly sauté the garlic and ginger.

9. Add the mushrooms and sauté together until tender.

10. Stir in the greens and sauté until all ingredients are completely mixed and heated.

11. Arrange the greens in a warmed serving dish and garnish with the cinnamon-flavored pine nuts.

## Julienned Beet and Carrot Slaw

The heart promotes the spleen and stomach. In Traditional Chinese Medicine, red foods help heart energy flow to the spleen and stomach. Yellow food for the spleen helps to continue that good energy flow (see Figure 1.2). The beets are especially good for your brain!

This dish is a perfect pairing of red and orange to promote good health.

## *Ingredients:*

- 1 red beet

- 1 carrot

- ½ teaspoon (2.5 ml) fresh ginger, minced

- 1 tablespoon of white sesame seeds

- 2 tablespoons (30 ml) freshly squeezed orange juice

- 2 teaspoons (10 ml) freshly squeezed lemon juice

- 2 teaspoons (10 ml) of extra virgin olive oil

- ¼ teaspoon (1.5 ml) Celtic sea salt

- 2 tablespoons chopped fresh Italian parsley.

## To Make:

1. Wash and peel the beet and carrot. Cut into thin, 2-inch x ¼-inch (5 cm by 1 cm) strips. Set aside in a serving dish.

2. In a small bowl, mix the minced ginger, white sesame seeds, juices, olive oil, and salt together.

3. Pour the liquid mixture over the beet and carrot pieces and toss together.

4. Garnish with parsley and serve.

# 15-minute Black Bean Salad

Try this salad recipe that only gets better with time. It is a great one to keep on hand in your refrigerator for a ready-made healthy meal or snack. Black beans strengthen the kidneys and help to clean your large intestines which is good for the brain.

## Ingredients

- 1/2 cup (75 g) finely chopped red onion

- 2 medium cloves, finely minced

- 2 cups (400 g) black beans or 1 15-oz can, drained and rinsed

- 1 cup (240 g) non-GMO frozen corn, thawed

- 8 cherry tomatoes, quartered

- 1/2 cup (90 g) coarsely chopped red pepper

- 2 tablespoons coarsely chopped pumpkin seeds

- 1/4 cup (15 g) chopped fresh Italian parsley

- 2 tablespoons (30 ml) extra virgin olive oil

- 3 (45 ml) tablespoons fresh lemon juice

- coarse Celtic sea salt and black pepper to taste

## *To make:*

1. Mince onions and garlic and let set for at least 5 minutes to bring out their health-promoting benefits.

2. Mix all ingredients together and serve. This salad will keep for a couple of days and gets more flavorful if you let it marinate in the refrigerator for a while.

Source: www.whfoods.com/genpage.php?tname=recipe&dbid=20.


# Black Cod Asian Style

(Requires marinating for a few hours.)
A deep cold water fish dish served up for your kidneys to love. A good source of iodine and selenium makes cod one of the healthiest fish dishes. Pistachios, a great source of energy, add an excellent source of vitamins and minerals.


## *Ingredients*

- 12 oz. (350 g) black cod steaks cut into 2 pieces

- ¼ cup (75 g) white miso

- ¼ cup (60 ml) sweet rice vinegar

- ¼ cup (60 ml) of saké or white cooking wine

- 1 tablespoon (15 ml) low sodium Tamari sauce

- 1 tablespoon (15 ml) maple syrup

- ½ cup coarsely chopped pistachio nuts


## *To Make:*

1. Add all liquid ingredients together in a pot and cook over a low heat. Stir until well mixed.

2. Place the cod in shallow baking dish, and pour the liquid over the filets.

3. Cover and refrigerate for a few hours or overnight.

4. When ready to cook the filets, preheat the oven to 425°F (220°C).

5. Before cooking, drain the filets to remove excess marinade.

6. Place the filets on a broiling pan and bake for 5 minutes or until glassy white and tender.

7. Then broil for 2 to 3 minutes to form a glaze on top.

8. Garnish with the chopped pistachio nuts.

9. Serve with a warm green vegetable dish.

## Honey and Maple Baked Pears

If your skin is feeling thirsty, try this dish to strengthen your lung function. Cherries, walnuts, honey, and cinnamon make it a complete natural healing dish.

### *Ingredients*

- 4 red Anjou or other variety of pears
- 3 tablespoons (45 g) unsalted butter, melted
- 2 tablespoons (60 g) local honey
- 2 tablespoons (30 ml) real maple syrup
- 3 teaspoons (15 ml) cinnamon
- ½ cup (50 g) raisins or chopped dried cherries
- ½ cup (60 g) coarsely chopped toasted walnuts.

### *To Make:*

1. Preheat the oven to 375° (190°).

2. Melt 2 tablespoons butter and coat the bottom and sides of a medium baking dish.

3. Wash the unpeeled pears, core, and chop into medium-sized cubes.

4. Arrange the cut pears in a baking dish.

5. Mix the honey, maple syrup, and half of the cinnamon together and drizzle over the pears.

6. Melt 1 tablespoon of butter in a small frying pan and sauté the walnuts and half of the cinnamon.

7. Sprinkle the raisins or dried cherries on top.

8. Sprinkle with buttered walnuts.

9. Bake at 375°F (190°C) for 15–20 minutes, or until the pears are tender.

For variety, you can substitute fresh, crisp apples for the pears.

## Buddha's Hand Vinegar from the NHRF

Buddha's hand vinegar combines the healing properties of vinegar with the healing benefits of the Buddha's hand fruit, a fruit with amazing health properties that is readily available in a dehydrated form. Buddha's hand vinegar may help to soothe the energy of the body, calm the mind, and improve your sleep. It is simply made by combining equal parts of juiced Buddha's hand fruit and reduced balsamic vinegar, and then diluting with water to taste and consistency. You can also add a pinch of Buddha's hand zest if desired and shake all the ingredients thoroughly together in a glass jar.

Enjoy 1–2 teaspoons a couple of times a day, or use as a dressing on a salad or sandwich. Add it to other juices or sparkling water for a refreshing drink. If you develop irritations in your mouth, dilute the mixture with water.

Buddha's hand vinegar has been used to relieve or improve stress, phlegm build-up, insomnia, depression, skin texture, stomach pain, and headaches. This citron fruit plays an important role in immune function due to its high vitamin C content (International Business Times 2014).

Fresh Buddha's hand fruit is usually available from November to January through online ordering. Also, look for it as a dried fruit throughout the year.

# About the Natural Healing Research Foundation (NHRF)

*Contributed by Dr. Lynn Thomas and Ann Yamamoto*

The Natural Healing Research Foundation, a 501(c)(3) non-profit organization, is dedicated to integrating proven natural healing practices with conventional medicine in a complementary way to augment treatment for global health issues. Grandmaster and his team established the foundation on June 7, 2004. The NHRF has a board of directors and designated officers who are entrusted to oversee the functions and operations of the foundation.

The foundation, with its main office in Hawaii, has become a valuable resource for natural healing methods to Hawaii's communities, as well as on the mainland. Dedicated volunteers have contributed thousands of hours to grow the foundation, obtain grants, expand community outreach, and utilize public relations and graphic/web design. Some of the volunteers have expanded their roles to become an integral part of the teacher team and the scientific research team. The instructors spent numerous hours teaching natural healing methods, medical Qigong exercises, and health-giving nutrition to the public and to specific populations. It was for the foundation's large and active Senior Program that Grandmaster developed a system of Exercises for the Aging Brain. Seniors are taught motivational exercises that are easy to do, yet effective in fighting and preventing a myriad of illnesses: heart disease, hypertension, chronic respiratory illness, diabetes, cancer, arthritis, dementia and other ailments common to an aging population. The program, funded by the NHRF, is offered to seniors at no cost.

As the NHRF grows, it offers an ever-expanding spectrum of health programs to people of all ages and capabilities. The foundation's year begins with the offering of a free Winter Immunity event to the community on the first of the three energetically coldest days of the year. Its companion event – Summer Respiratory – takes place on the first of the three energetically hottest days and is also a charitable event. These two seminars are unique in that, in addition to sharing many natural healing methods, they provide free herbal patches which are placed on specific points of the body to aid the body's respective immune and respiratory systems.

Through an alliance with the Partners in Development Foundation (FID), the NHRF participates in outreach programs such as Tutu, Qi and Me, which teaches natural healing exercises for children and their elders/grandparents to do together – a winning combination that benefits both generations.

The Foundation is now developing a free program for retired United States military veterans and their immediate families to address the issues that continue to plague returning combat soldiers: Post Traumatic Syndrome Disorders (PTSD), exposure to Agent Orange, drug abuse, and other psychological and psychiatric traumas. This program integrates natural healing Qigong exercises with expressions of sounds, rejuvenating foods and beverages, all ending with a moment of meditative silence.

Throughout the year, the foundation hosts workshops on a variety of health subjects that incorporate natural healing and Traditional Chinese Medicine methods. The community continues to benefit from workshops and seminars on subjects such as cancer, diabetes, heart disease and hypertension, ADD and ADHD, inflammation, weight loss, arthritis, gout, liver diseases, Chronic Fatigue Syndrome, stress, female health and fertility, insomnia, better vision practices, aging and longevity – including NHRF's Exercises for the Aging Brain, improving musical ability, the Body Pyramid® exercise system, and infant and toddler healing massages. The NHRF also hosts retreats for teacher trainings and personal wellness. It has held two highly successful pilot drug rehabilitation programs. The events and retreats have highlighted the importance of strengthening the mind, body, and spirit while providing the simple means to do so.

By sharing the practices of Qigong, Traditional Chinese Medicine and natural healing with communities, and with the larger public, the Natural Healing Research Foundation is fulfilling Grandmaster's original mission in a much larger scope than would have ever been possible for one man from China.

**Thanks to the following foundation members, as well as many anonymous donors, who have made the Senior Wellness Program possible:**

Joyce Settle – Foundation co-founder

Scott Galper – Translator, Program office

Dr. Lynn Thomas – Program office

Wade Shigemasa – Head instructor

Millannie Mattson – Program teacher

Pua Kekina – Senior wellness coordinator and program teacher

Jimmy Kekina – Program teacher

Ann Yamamoto – Qi Center, Honolulu coordinator

Stephanie Eggert – Program office

Amina Khan-Miyasaki – Translator, Program office

Chablis Paris – Website design and public relations

Miriam Miyai – Program office

Mae Klein – Program teacher

Irene Au – Program teacher

Erin Mattson – Program teacher

Michael Bacaro – Program teacher

Arlene Wong – Program assistant

Joy Tanabe – Program teacher

Ruby Yuen – Program assistant

Keren Siket – Foundation vice president

Kathleen and JC Coelho – Program teachers

Kathie Ong – Program teacher

Evans and Barbara Yim – Qi Center site donors

Mark Siket – Program teacher

Joan Stone – Program teacher

# References

Brain Injury Research Institute (2009) *4 Exercises to Sharpen Your Brain*. Wheeling, WV: Brain Injury Institute, Inc. Accessed on 23 Sept 2014 at www.ij-cm.org/4-exercises-to-sharpen-your-brain.php.

Cassels, C. (2013) *Novel Exercise Program May Trump Meds for Dementia*. New York, NY: Medscape News from WebMD. Accessed on 13 April 2013 at www.Medscape.com/viewarticle/781607.

Doctors Health Press Editorial Board (2005) *FDA Warns Antipsychotics May Increase Death in Seniors*. Boston, MA: Doctors Health Press. Accessed on 30 Jan 2013 at www.doctorshealthpress.com/brain-function-articles/fda-warns-antipsychotics-may-increase-death-in-seniors.

Doctors Health Press Editorial Board (2011a) *Alzheimer's May be Detectable Years before Onset*. Boston, MA: Doctors Health Press. Accessed on 30 Jan 2013 at www.doctorshealthpress.com/brain-function-%20 articles/alzheimers-may-be-detectable-years-before-onset.

Doctors Health Press Editorial Board (2011b) *Laughter Helps Keep Alzheimer's Symptoms Away*. Boston, MA: Doctors Health Press. Accessed on 24 Feb 2013 at www.doctorshealthpress.com/food-and-nutrition-articles/laughter-helps-keep-alzheimers-symptoms-away.

Edelson, E. (2006) *Brain's Oxygen Supply Key to Alzheimer's Risk*. Washington, DC: The Washington Post. Accessed on 1 Aug 2013 at www.washingtonpost.com/wp-dyn/content/article/2006/11/20/AR2006112000835.html.

Harvard Women's Health Watch (2009) 'The Health Benefits of Tai Chi.' *Harvard Women's Health Watch 16*, 9, 2-4.

Health Realizations (2013) *Research Shows You Can Worry Yourself Into Dementia and Even Alzheimer's*. Beverly Hills, CA: Khalsa Medical Clinic. Accessed on 1 April 2014 at http://articles.healthrealizations. com/KhalsaMedicalClinic/2013/05/27/Research-Now-Shows-You-Can-Worry-Yourself-1. aspx?SubscriberEmail=ariannahuf@huffingtonpost.com.

Humphreys, I. (2009) *Immunity in the Salivary Gland*. London: British Society for Immunology. Accessed on 28 Sept 2014 at www.bitesized.immunology.org/organs-and-tissues/immunity-in-the-salivary-gland.

International Business Times (2014) *Buddha's Hand: Fruit for Good Luck, Happiness and Long Life*. Australian Edition: International Business Times. Accessed on 13 Nov 2014 at http://au.ibtimes.com/articles/ 546150/20140402/buddha-s-hand-fruit-diet-healthy-fitness.htm#.VgutQL4b81A.

Lee, M., Lee, M. S., Kim, H., Choi, E. (2004) 'Effects of Qigong on Blood Pressure, High-density Lipoprotein Cholesterol and Other Lipid Levels in Essential Hypertensive Patients.' *International Journal of Neuroscience 114*, 7, 777–786.

Liu, H. with Perry, P. (1997) *The Healing Art of Qi Gong*. New York, NY: Warner Books.

Lu, N. with Schaplowsky E. (2000) *Traditional Chinese Medicine: A Natural Guide to Weight Loss That Lasts*. New York, NY: Harper Collins.

Lui, W., Gong, C. (2009) *Expert Advice: Treatment of Seasonal Disorders – Spring in Traditional Chinese Medicine*. Roseville, MN: TCMpage. Accessed on 29 July 2012 at www.tcmpage.com/spring_disorders.html.

Maoshing, N. (2009) "4 exercises to sharpen your brain." Accessed on 28 March 2014 at http://health. yahoo.com/experts/drmao/19035/4-exercises-to-sharpen-your-brain.

Marchione, V. (2011) *New Cause of Memory Loss Discovered*. Boston, MA: Doctors Health Press. Accessed on 2 Feb 2013 at www.doctorshealthpress.com/brain-function-articles/memory-articles/new-cause-of-memory-loss-discovered.

Marchione, V. (2012) *Your Hands and Feet Could Predict Dementia.* Boston, MA: Doctors Health Press. Accessed on 29 Feb 2013 at www.doctorshealthpress.com/brain-function-articles/your-hands-and-feet-could-predict-dementia.

Marichione, M. (2011) *Alzheimer's Debate: Test If You Can't Treat It?* McLean, VA: USA Today. Accessed on 26 Feb 2013 at www.usatoday30.usatoday.com/news/health/medical/health/medical/alzheimers/story/2011/07/Alzheimers-debate-Test-if-you-cant-treat-it/49576628/1.

Morelli, J., Chang, L. (2014) *What Are the Side Effects of Allergy Medications.* New York, NY: RxList owned by WebMD. Accessed on 23 Sept 2014 at www.rxlist.com/allergy_medications-page3/drugs-condition.htm.

National Institute of Health (2012) *Anemia in Chronic Kidney Disease.* The National Kidney and Urologic Disease Information Clearinghouse (NKUDIC) Fact Sheet. Bethesda MD: NIH Accessed on 30 June 2012 at http://kidney.niddk.nih.gov/kudiseases/pubs/anemia/anemia_508.pdf.

Pacific College of Oriental Medicine (PCOM) (2014) *Emotions and Traditional Chinese Medicine.* San Diego, CA: PCOM. Accessed on 14 Nov 2014 at www.pacificcollege.edu?acupuncture-massage-news/articles/448-emotions-and-traditional-chinese-medicine.html.

Poole, J. (2008) *The Be-In-Better-Balance-Book.* Watertown, MA: Pooled Resources.

Renneboog, B., Musch, W., Vandermergel, X., *et al.* (2006) 'Mild Chronic Hyponatremia is Assoiated with Falls, Unsteadiness, and Attention Deficits.' *The American Journal of Medicine* 119, 6, 71–78.

Sacks, F. (2014) *Ask the Expert: Omega-3 Fatty Acids.* Boston, MA: The Nutrition Source, Harvard School of Public Health. Accessed on 24 Sept 2014 at www.hsph.harvard.edu/nutritionsource/omega-3.

Sancier, K. (1996) *Anti-Aging Benefits of Qigong.* Los Altos, CA: The Qigong Institute. Accessed on 30 May 2012 at www.qigonginstitute.org/html/papers/Anti-Aging_Benefits_of_Qigong.html.

Sancier, K. (1999). 'Therapeutic Benefits of Qigong Exercises in Combination with Drugs.' *Journal of Alternative and Complementary Medicine 5,* 4, 383–389.

Scripps Research Institute (2011) *Liver, not brain, may be origin of Alzheimer's plaques.* ScienceDaily. Retrieved 18 January 2015 from www.sciencedaily.com/releases/2011/03/110303134435.htm

Seligson, M.R., (1995-2013) Caregiver Burnout. Fort Lauderdale, FL: Caregiver Media Group. Accessed on 10 Jan 2013 at www.caregiver.com/articles/caregiver/caregiver_burnout.htm

Semel Institute, UCLA (2013) *The Biopsychosocial Outcomes of Mindful Exercise and Meditation Used for Treatment and Prevention of Mental Disorders.* Los Angles, CA: Jane & Terry Semel Institute for Neuroscience & Human Behavior. Accessed on 24 Aug 2014 at www.semel.ucla.edu/latelife/blog/hlavretsuclaedu/biopsychosocial-outcomes-mindful-exercise-meditation-used-treatment-pr.

Shah, R., (2013) *Wise Food Choices May Delay Alzheimer's Disease Development and Progression.* Solon, OH: Nutrition Remarks. Accessed on 24 Sept 2014 at www.nutritionremarks.com/?s=omega+3+dha.

Sheikh, J. (2010) "Allergy medicine: 8 surprising possible side effects. (PHOTOS)." *The Huffington Post* (24 November). Accessed on 13 April 2014 at www.huffingtonpost.com/2010/11/24/allergy-medicine-surprisin_n_787559.html#s190139title=Low_Libido.

Shen-Nong (2006a) *How Does TCM View Obesity and Its Causes?* Hong Kong: Integrated Chinese Medical Holdings, Ltd. Accessed on 5 Dec 2012 at: www.shen-nong.com/eng/lifestyles/tcmrole_obesityweight_cause.html.

Shen-Nong (2006b) *What Are the Yin Yang Organs?* Hong Kong: Integrated Chinese Medical Holdings, Ltd. Accessed on 5 Dec 2012 at www.shen-nong.com/eng/principles/whatyinyangorgans.html.

Smith, M., Russell, D., White, M. (2013) Alzheimer's Behavior Management – Managing Symptoms: Wandering. Santa Monica, CA USA: Helpguide.org International. Accessed on 3 Mar 2013 at http://www.helpguide.org/elder/alzheimers_behavior_problems.htm.

TCM Student (2005) *Functions of the Liver.* Philadelphia, PA: Philadelphia Acupuncture, LLC. Accessed on 5 Sept 2013 at www.tcmstudent.com/theory/Function%20Liver.html.

TCM World Foundation (2014) *The Dragon's Way Recipes for Self-healing.* New York, NY: TCM World Foundation. Accessed on 29 Sept 2014 at www.tcmworld.org/dragonsway/the-dragons-way-recipes-for-self-healing.

University of Chicago Medicine (2005) Enriched Environment Delays Onset of Alzheimer's in Mice. Chicago, IL: The University of Chicago Medicine. Accessed on 23 Feb 2013 at www.uchospitals.edu/news/2005/20050311-alzheimers.html

Wayne, P. and Fuerst, M. (2013) *The Harvard Medical School Guide to Tai Chi.* Boston, MA: Shambhala Publications.

WebMD (2009) *Digestive Disorders Health Center, Picture of the Liver.* New York, NY: WebMD Ltd. Accessed on 5 Sept 2013 at www.webmd.com/digestive-disorders/picture-of-the-liver.

WebMD (2009) *Incontinence & Overactive Bladder Health.* New York, NY: WebMD Ltd. Accessed on 12 January 2015 at http://www.webmd.com/urinary-incontinence-oab/picture-of-the-kidneys

Wiley's Supper Club (2014) *The Color of Health.* Fairfield, CT: Uncle Wiley's, Inc. Accessed on 25 Sept 2014 at www.unclewileys.com/index.php/content/view/42/40.

Windblad, L. (2010) *Foods for Good Nerves and Veins.* Chicago, IL: Diet Health Club of Everyday Health, Inc. Accessed on 13 Nov 2014 at www.diethealthclub.com/articles/491/diet-and-wellness/foods-good-for-nerves-and-veins.html.

World Tai Chi & Qigong Day (2005) *Exercise Helps Reduce Alzheimer's Onset.* Overland Park, KS: World Tai Chi & Qigong Day. Accessed on 16 June 2012 at www.worldtaichiday.org/ALZHEIMERSDISEASE. html.

World's Healthiest Foods, The (2014) *15 Minute Black Bean Salad.* Glendale, CA: The George Mateljan Foundation. Accessed on 1 Jan. 2015 at www.whfoods.com/genpage.php?tname=biosketch&dbid=3

Yi, D. (2006) *What Are the Energies, Flavors and Other Properties of Foods?* Hong Kong: Shen-Nong of Integrated Chinese Medical Holdings, Ltd. Accessed 5 Dec 2012 at www.shen-nong.com/eng/ lifestyles/food_property_food_tcm.html.

Yin Yang House (2011) *How I Love the Meridian Clock or Meridian Flow Wheel.* Chattanooga, TN USA: Yin Yang House. Accessed on 29 July 2012 at http://www.yinyanghouse.com/practitioner_members/ general-energywork/how-i-love-meridian-clock-or-meridian-flow-wheel.

# Further Reading

Bardot, J. (2012) 'To every food there is a season, color, taste, element. Your organs know this, do you?' *Natural News*. Accessed on 25 August 2014 at www.naturalnews.com/036876_five_elements_food_seasons.html.

Black, D. S., Cole, S. W., Irwin, M. R., *et al.* (2013) 'Yogic Meditation Reverses NF-kappaB and IRF-related Transcriptome Dynamics in Leukocytes of Family Dementia Caregivers in a Randomized Controlled Trial.' *Psychoneuroendocrinology 38*, 3, 348–355.

Chiesa, A., Serretti A. (2010) 'A Systematic Review of Neurobiological and Clinical Features of Mindfulness Meditations.' *Psychological Medicine 40*, 8, 1039–1052.

Easton, J. (2005) *Enriched Environment Reduced Alzheimer's Dangerous Peptides in Mice.* Chicago, IL: The University of Chicago Chronicle 24, 12. Accessed on 23 Feb 2013 at www.chronicle.uchicago.edu/050317/alzheimers.shtml.

Feil, Naomi (1993) *The Validation Breakthrough.* Baltimore, MD: Health Professionals Press.

Horrigan, B. (2005) 'Meditation and Neuroplasticity: Training Your Brain' (Interview with Richard Davidson, Ph.D). *Explore 1*, 381–388.

Karsten, S., Geschwind, D. (2005) 'Exercise Your Amyloid.' *Cell 120*, 11 Mar 2005, 572–574.

Lavretsky, H., Epel, E. S., Siddarth, P., *et al.* (2013) 'A Pilot Study of Yogic Meditation for Family Dementia Caregivers with Depressive Symptoms: Effects on Mental Health, Cognition, and Telomerase Activity.' *International Journal of Geriatric Psychiatry 28*, 1, 57–65.

Lazarov, O., Robinson, J., Tang, Y., Sisodia, S., *et al.* (2005) 'Environmental Enrichment Reduces Aβ Levels and Amyloid Deposition in Transgenic Mice.' *Cell 120*, 11 Mar 2005, 701–713.

Myung, S. L., Myeong S. L., Hye-Jung, K., and Euy-Soon, C. (2004) 'Effects of QiGong on blood pressure, high-density lipoprotein cholesterol and other lipid levels in essential hypertensive patients.' *International Journal of Neuroscience 114*, 7, 777–786. Accessed on 19 April 2013 at http://informahealthcare.com.

Ni, Mao Shing (2012) *Dr. Mao's Secrets of Longevity Cookbook.* Kansas City, MO: Andrews McMeel Publishing.

Pomykala, K., Silverman, D., Geist, C., *et al.* (2012) 'A Pilot Study of the Effects of Meditation on Regional Brain Metabolism in Distressed Dementia Caregivers.' *Aging Health 8*, 5, 509–516.

Shen-Nong (2006) *What Are the Seven Emotions.* Hong Kong: Integrated Chinese Medical Holdings, Ltd. Accessed on 20 Nov 2014 at www.shen-nong.com/eng/principles/sevenemotions.html.

Shih, Tzu Kuo (1994) *Qi Gong Therapy: the Chinese Art of Healing with Energy.* New York: Station Hill Press

Slagter, H. *et al.* (2011) 'Mental Training as a Tool in the Neuroscientific Study of Brain and Cognitive Plasticity.' *Frontiers in Neuroscience Research 5*, 17.

Sun, X., He, G., Qing, H., Song, W., *et al.* (2006) 'Hypoxia Facilitates Alzheimer's Disease Pathogenesis by Up-regulationg BACE1 Gene Expression.' *Proceedings of the National Academy of Sciences 103*, 49, 18727–18732.

Tooley, G. A., Armstrong, S. M., Norman, T. R., Sali, A. (2000) 'Acute Increases in Night-time Plasma Melatonin Levels Following a Period of Meditation.' *Biological Psychology 53*, 1, 69–78.

Voelcker-Rehage, C. and Willimczik, K. (2006) 'Motor Plasticity in a Juggling Task in Older Adults – A Developmental Study.' *Age and Ageing 35*, 4, 422–427.

Wayne, P. with Fuerst, M. (2013) *Harvard Medical School Guide to Tai Chi*, p.282. Boston, MA: Shambhala Publications.

Wei, L. and Changzhen, C. (2009) "Chinese Medicine for Your Disorders in Spring Season." *Traditional Chinese Medicine Information Page*. Accessed on 24 August 2014 at www.tcmpage.com/spring_disorders.html.

Wilson, R., Schneider, J., Boyle, P., Arnold, S., *et al.* (2007) 'Chronic Distress and Incidence of Mild Cognitive Impairment.' *Neurology 68*, 2085–2092.

Wu, E., Barnes, D. E., Ackerman, S. L., Lee, J., Chesney, M., Mehling, W. E. (2014) *Preventing Loss of Independence Through Exercise (PLIÉ): Qualitative Analysis of a Clinical Trial in Older Adults with Dementia in Aging & Mental Health*. London, UK: Taylor & Francis for Routledge Informa Ltd. Accessed on 24 Sept 2013 at www.dx.doi.org/10.1080/13607863.2014.935290.

Wu, Zong and Mao, Li (eds) (1992) *Ancient Way to Keep Fit*. Bolinas, CA: Shelter Publications. (Original work published 1990).

**The following are suggested readings on the topic of the brain:**
*Among reported changes in human studies are higher levels of cerebral blood flow and blood volume*
Rogers, R. L. *et al.* (1990) 'After Reaching Retirement Age Physical Activity Sustains Cerebral Perfusion and Cognition.' *Journal of the American Geriatrics Society 38*, 2, 123–28.

Periera, A. C. *et al.* (2007) 'An in Vivo Correlate of Exercise-induced Neurogenesis in the Adult Dentate Gyrus.' *Proceedings of the National Academy of Sciences of the United States of America 104*, 113, 5638–43.

*Increased activity in frontal and parietal regions of the brain, which are thought to be involved in efficient attentional control*
Colcombe, S. J. *et al.* (2004) 'Cardiovascular Fitness, Cortical Plasticity, and Aging.' *Proceedings of the National Society of Sciences of the United States of America 101*, 9, 3316–21. *Increased gray and white matter volume in the prefrontal cortex*

Colcombe S. J. *et al.* (2006) 'Aerobic Exercise Training Increases Brain Volume in Aging Humans.' *Journals of Gerontology Series A: Biological Sciences and Medical Sciences 61*, 11, 1166–70.

*An increased functioning of key nodes in the brain's executive control*
Watson *et al.* (2010) 'Executive Function, Memory, and Gait Speed Decline in Well-functioning Older Adults.' *Journals of Gerontology Series A: Biological Sciences and Medical Sciences 65*, 1093–100.

*Default networks*
Voss, M. W. *et al.* (2010) 'Plasticity of Brain Networks in a Randomized Intervention Trial of Exercise Training in Older Adults.' *Frontiers in Aging Neuroscience 26*, 2, 316.

# Index

Smith, M. 48
sound therapy 59, 69, 94–100
spleen 28–9
    associations
        animal 68, 98
        Earth 17–8, 62
        emotion 44, 54, 94, 98
        paired organ 49
        season and color 68
        taste 136
    exercises for 98, 124–5, 127
    food for 136–7, 140–1,
        146–7, 150–1
    interdependence of organs
        31, 67
    location of points 102
    as main producer of Qi 30
    responsibility 16
spring onions 142
stagnation 17, 31, 69
stomach
    associations
        animal 95, 98
        Earth 17, 62
        emotion 44, 94, 98
        paired organ 49
        season, color and taste
            136
    exercises for 98, 111, 126–7
    food for 137, 140–4,
        146–7, 150–1, 154
    interdependence of organs
        30–1
    location of points 102
    responsibility 17
Stomp and Clap to Move
    Energy Throughout Your
    Body 91
strawberries 142
stress 51, 61–2, 70–1, 101,
    154
strokes 32, 39–41
"sundown syndrome" 14, 48–9,
    65, 68
superoxide dismutase (SOD)
    30, 42
Swallowing Saliva in Thirds for
    Good Digestion 127–8, 131

T'ai Chi 14–5, 20, 37, 51
Tap the Inner Edges of Your
    Hands-Palms Facing Away 79
Tap the Outer Edges of Your
    Hands-Palms Facing You 78

Tap Your Finger Tips to Move
    Your Energy 77–8
TCM Student 30
TCM World Foundation 146
thyroid gland, exercise for 114
tiger
    associations 68, 95
    exercise 96
    healing sounds of 54, 59
tongue exercise 121–2, 130
Traditional Chinese Medicine
    (TCM) 16–7
    auditory perception and
        kidney functioning 47
    color of foods 69–70
    on formation of disease 25
    on function of spleen 28
    interdependence of organs
        31–3
    organs and emotions 43–4,
        58
    perspective on dementia
        23–5, 67
    perspective on diet 135–6
    "you are what you eat" adage
        135
Traditional Chinese Medicine
    Education Center of Canada
    137
Triple Heater 127
Twelve Sitting Exercises
    117–31
twenty-four hour cycle of
    energy 66–7

University of Chicago Medicine
    37

walnuts 70, 137–8, 140, 142,
    145, 151–2
Warm Greens Mix-Up 149–50
Warm Up Your Energy 77
Warming Your Kidneys for
    Longevity 122–3, 130
Wash Your Face With Energy
    103
Water
    corresponding emotion,
        season, animal and color
        68
    corresponding organs 17–8
watermelon 140, 142
Wayne, P. 15, 51
WebMD 29

Western perspectives 14–5,
    18–9, 23–33, 57–8, 69–71
Wiley's Supper Club 69
White, M. 48
whole being 18–19
Windblad, L. 138
Wipe the Old Energy from Your
    Chin 113
Wood
    corresponding emotion,
        season, animal and color
        68
    corresponding organs 17–8
World Tai Chi and Qigong Day
    37, 59
worry
    as afflictive emotion 54
    associations
        animal 95, 98
        element 18
        organ 44, 94
        season and color 68
        taste 136
    as contributing to
        development of dementia
        10, 53
    exercise for 98
    as sign of spleen dysfunction
        28

Yank Gently on Your Ears to
    Awaken the Energy Deep
    Inside 108
Yi, D. 135
yin and yang 16–7, 66–8, 135
Yin Meditation to Build Energy
    128–9, 131
Yin-Yang Feet to Balance Your
    Energy 90

Zhu Xilin, Master 10

zucchini 142

CPI Antony Rowe
Eastbourne, UK
June 20, 2023

# Skills Guidance

## ■ Practical advice

### Following written procedures

When carrying out practical work you usually follow a set of written instructions. Before you start the practical work read these through to the end. Annotate the instructions to help you understand them. Then check that you have all the apparatus and materials listed. When you are ready to start, read the first instruction carefully and carry it out. Put a tick by each instruction when you have completed it. Proceed carefully through the rest of the instructions, double-checking that you are sticking to them. This is important to ensure the collection of accurate data and to make the practical activity safe. Following instructions shows competency in CPAC 1.

### Investigative approaches

You may be asked to plan an aspect of an investigation in the exam papers and you will probably plan and carry out a complete investigation as part of your practical work so that you can be assessed on your investigative approach for CPAC 2.

Throughout your course and in the examinations you will be tested on the skills involved in planning, such as identifying variables, stating a hypothesis, writing a method or explaining how to collect results and/or analyse them. Writing full plans during your course will prepare you well for these questions. Here are some steps to follow while planning an investigation:

1 **Identify a question to answer and write a hypothesis**. Read the information provided and look for clues. Write a question that you have to answer by experiment and then write a hypothesis, which is a clear statement about what you think will happen. You must write a **testable hypothesis** — one that you can test by experiment.

2 **Carry out some research**. Use sources of information to read about the problem you are trying to solve. Look for ideas to help your planning and decide how results will be analysed statistically.

3 **Write a null hypothesis**. If you are going to use a statistical test to analyse your results then you must rewrite your hypothesis as a negative statement, known as a **null hypothesis**. This states the opposite of your hypothesis. Your experiment must test the idea that there will be *no effect*.

4 **Identify the independent, dependent and control variables for the investigation:**
   - **Independent variable** (IV) — the variable you change.
   - **Dependent variable** (DV) — the variable you measure or observe.
   - **Control variables** (CV) — the variables that are kept constant, because they might affect the values of the DV.

5 **Decide on a strategy for your experiment**. This is a brief outline of a method that tests your hypothesis.

6 **Choose apparatus and materials that are appropriate**. You should be able to select appropriate equipment to collect accurate data. Often it is a good idea to justify your choice of the main items of apparatus. An important consideration is the resolution of the apparatus you use.

**Resolution** is the smallest change in quantity that can be measured with the apparatus that you are using. This refers both to the apparatus used to measure out quantities as part of the procedure and the apparatus used to collect results. It refers to the number of significant figures (or decimal places) in readings.

When measuring out volumes, for example, you might use a syringe, pipette, burette or measuring cylinder. A burette measures to the nearest $0.1\,cm^3$ so you would select a burette if you were measuring $0.5\,cm^3$ of a solution, but this resolution would not be necessary if you wanted to measure $100\,cm^3$.

When collecting results, a balance might weigh to the nearest $0.1\,g$; some balances are more sensitive and weigh to the nearest $0.01\,g$. If measuring change in length you would use a ruler that measures to the nearest millimetre. These are measures of resolution in results taking. Recording to the nearest $0.01\,g$ gives a higher resolution than measuring to $0.1\,g$. Similarly, measuring to the nearest millimetre gives a higher resolution than measuring to the nearest centimetre. In this context resolution means the number of significant figures or decimal places to which values are expressed.

Stop clocks and bench timers can often measure to a hundredth of a second ($0.01\,s$). It is highly unlikely that you could time a colour change or other event to this degree of resolution, so it is better to express such results to the nearest second.

7 **Expand the strategy into a detailed procedure, using numbered steps**. Avoid using continuous prose — it is easier to follow a series of instructions. Notice that numbered points allow you to include instructions such as 'repeat step 6'. The procedure must describe how results are to be collected.

8 **Explain how results are to be presented**. A good way to do this is to draw a table with clear column headings, including units.

9 **Explain how results are to be analysed**. This includes:
   - data processing
   - graphs
   - statistical tests

10 **Plan and carry out a preliminary investigation** to trial your ideas. You may have to modify your procedure as a result. If so, record the modifications you made and why you made them in your report.

**Practical tip**

If you choose to use a colorimeter, you could say that this gives quantitative results that are easier for others to reproduce than if you use colour standards (charts showing expected colours). You will use a colorimeter in required practical 11.

**Practical tip**

Notice that resolution also applies to microscopy. It refers to the smallest distance that can be detected when using a microscope.

# Safety

Planning and carrying out practical work safely is essential and demonstrates competency in CPAC 3. If you work unsafely, you are not only putting yourself at risk, but also other people in the class.

A risk assessment should be completed before any practical activity is undertaken. The responsibility for this lies with your school or college, but you may be asked to write a risk assessment for one or more of the required practicals. Your school or college should have documents on safety published by an organisation known as CLEAPSS (Consortium of Local Education Authorities for the Provision of Science Services) that you could refer to for details of possible risks and how to control them.

The following is some general safety advice, but if you are unsure of something, it is important that you check with your teacher.

- Keep your work area well organised and tidy.
- Use one area for wet work and keep another area dry for writing your notes. Do your practical work over the bench, not over your papers.
- Wear protective goggles/spectacles when using liquids or when cutting anything.
- Make sure that you are familiar with hazard warning symbols and know how to respond to them.
- Take special care when using knives, scalpels, glassware, chemicals, Bunsen flames, hot water etc.
- Inform the teacher or technician immediately if you have an accident.
- Clear up any spillages or broken glass immediately.

Table 1 shows examples of poor laboratory practice, together with equivalent good practice.

**Practical tip**

Your teacher will assess your approach to working methodically and safely while you carry out your practical work.

**Practical tip**

Syringes should be washed out with water and then with a small volume of the liquid that you are going to dispense.

**Table 1** Examples of poor and good laboratory practice

| Poor practice | Good practice |
|---|---|
| Using incorrect apparatus or equipment without realising*, for example using a $10\,cm^3$ syringe instead of a $1\,cm^3$ to dispense $0.5\,cm^3$ of a liquid | Choosing the correct apparatus/equipment/chemicals from those provided so that the correct results are obtained |
| Using the same syringe to dispense different liquids without realising* so that contamination occurs | Using separate syringes when necessary and keeping syringes separate once used (for correct re-use) or washing out a syringe between using to dispense different solutions |
| Cutting slices or cubes or sections carelessly so that sections are of uneven thickness or cubes are of unequal size | Using cutting equipment (e.g. scalpels and knives) and measuring equipment (e.g. rulers) with care to produce slices and cubes of correct sizes |
| Allowing fluids to drip off the outside of beakers/tubing/stirring rods/tissue samples into other solutions so that there is the risk of cross-contamination | Rinsing and drying equipment when necessary, clearing off spills on the outside of beakers; keeping different items in clearly defined areas on the bench |
| Haphazard use of the stop clock/bench timer so that incorrect times are recorded; samples are not taken at correct time intervals | Checking how to use the stop clock/bench timer before starting; careful checking of times; re-setting back to zero when required |
| Filtering suspensions through a filter funnel where the filter paper has not been folded correctly/has a tear/has not been fitted into the funnel correctly | Folding a piece of filter paper and then opening it out into the filter funnel; filtering suspensions so that a clear solution, the filtrate, runs through and the precipitate/larger insoluble particles remain on the filter paper |

* Realising a mistake and asking for fresh syringes is considered good practice.

# Recording observations

Making accurate observations and recording them in a suitable form is an important skill that provides evidence for CPAC 4. In most cases, results and observations will be recorded in tables.

Before you start to draw a table, decide what you need to record. Decide on how many columns and how many rows you will need. Make sure you have read all the practical instructions before you draw the table outline. Follow these rules:

- The first column should be the independent variable, the second and subsequent columns should contain the dependent variables.
- Write clear and detailed headings for each column.
- The headings of the columns must include the relevant units. There should be no units in the body of the table.

**Practical tip**

Units are separated from the description of the variable by a forward slash (/). The slash should *not* be used to mean 'per' in compound units. For example, do *not* write g per $cm^3$ as g/$cm^3$, but as $g\,cm^{-3}$.

- Data should be ordered so that trends and patterns can be seen — it is best to arrange the values of the independent variable in ascending order.
- Use plenty of space — do not make the table too small.
- Leave some space to the right of the table in case you decide you need to add more columns.
- Use a pencil and ruler to draw lines between the columns and between the rows. Rule lines around the whole table.

# Evaluating procedures

A sound understanding of the required practicals is essential, so a thorough analysis of your results will prepare you for the exams as well as providing evidence for CPAC 5. When evaluating an experimental procedure it is important to consider the way in which the procedure was carried out and the quality of the data collected. You need to ask yourself the question: 'can I have confidence in my data?' If you do not have confidence in the data then you cannot have confidence in the conclusion(s) that you make.

The first thing to do when evaluating is to consider the procedure that you followed. Is it possible that there were any **measurement errors** in the method? There are two types of error:

- **Systematic errors** are always the same throughout the investigation. A common type of systematic error is that the measuring device may give readings that are incorrect by a certain value. It could be that one of the control variables is always incorrect by the same quantity. If there are small systematic errors (that are always the same) then the data may be precise, but not accurate. The effect of these errors is to overestimate or underestimate the true values of the dependent variable.

**Practical tip**

There are plenty of examples in this guide to help you become proficient in drawing and completing tables of results.

**Practical tip**

The general rules for drawing tables apply whether producing a hand-drawn table in your lab book, or using a spreadsheet program.

**Practical tip**

Never jot your results down on pieces of rough paper. Draw a table to record your raw data in your lab book so that you can refer back to it if necessary.

**Practical tip**

The words in **bold** type are important key terms that you must understand and use. Look for the use of these terms in the Questions & Answers section.

- **Random errors** occur when you do not carry out the procedure in exactly the same way each time. You may also read the apparatus in a slightly different way each time you take a reading. These errors affect some of the results, but not all of them. They do not always affect the results in the same way. Random errors could be the result of the variation in biological material.

Do not think of errors as mistakes. Even in a perfectly conducted investigation, there will be errors.

You should consider the control variables involved in the investigation. These should be kept constant, or monitored if it is not possible to keep them constant. If these variables are not controlled then they may influence the results; they are called **confounding variables** or **uncontrolled variables**. Sometimes, particularly in fieldwork studies when you cannot control certain abiotic factors, you may be aware of such variables and then 'take them into account' when analysing and interpreting results.

Control variables should not be confused with a **control experiment**. A control experiment is important to show that your results are valid. For example, if you are investigating the effect of temperature on the hydrolysis of starch by amylase, you need to show that it is the amylase that is causing the hydrolysis rather than the buffer solution or heat. A control experiment may involve using boiled amylase to show that hydrolysis is due to enzyme action.

There are several terms with specific meanings that are used when discussing the quality of the procedure and the results obtained:

- **Accuracy** is a measure of how close a result is to an accepted 'true' value. In biological investigations the true value is not always known. In some cases results can be checked with sources of data. For example, tidal volume readings should be about $500\,cm^3$, the water potential of the blood should be equivalent to 0.9% sodium chloride solution ($-3.86\,MPa$), but the water potential of plant tissues varies considerably and there is no specific value against which results can be checked.
- **Anomalous results** are results that do not fit the trend. They can be:
  - replicate results that differ significantly from others
  - results for one value of the independent variable that do not fit the overall trend

> **Practical tip**
>
> Anomalous results should not be ignored. You should initially repeat the result and see if you get a similar reading. If you do, you should then consider possible causes; for example:
> - Is the solution from the same batch?
> - Is it due to experimental error?
> - Have you used a different piece of measuring equipment?

- **Precision** is a measure of the closeness of agreement between individual results obtained using the same procedure under exactly the same conditions. However, closeness of replicates does not mean that the data are close to the true value.
- **Repeatable results** are replicate results that are in close agreement. You can use mathematical methods to help evaluate the variation in replicate results. In A-level practical tasks it is usual to carry out three repeats or replicates for each value of

**Accuracy** refers to how close a measurement is to its true value.

> **Practical tip**
>
> Take special care not to overuse the term accuracy. There are very few biology investigations when you can say what the true value(s) should be.

**Precision** refers to the spread of measurements about the mean value.

> **Practical tip**
>
> Calculating a **running mean** is a good way to check that you have enough replicate results. Calculate the mean after you have collected each replicate and continue doing this until it remains near constant.

the independent variable if time and materials permit. These should be carried out separately from each other, using exactly the same experimental procedures.

- Results are **reproducible** if someone else who repeats the investigation obtains the same results as you. You can only comment on this in response to a question if you are given results from another person.

- **Uncertainty** is half the smallest graduation on the apparatus. For example, if the smallest division on a syringe is $1.0\,cm^3$ then the uncertainty would be $\pm 0.5\,cm^3$. If you are certain that you have started measuring at 0, then the uncertainty applies where you take the measurement, so $6.3\,cm^3$ is expressed as $6.3 \pm 0.5\,cm^3$. If you are not sure that you started measuring exactly at 0 or you have started at a measurement other than 0 (for example when using a burette) the uncertainty applies at both ends, so it is multiplied by two as there is an error at each end, giving an uncertainty of $\pm 1.0\,cm^3$.

  It is possible to calculate the **percentage error** for the apparatus you used for measuring your results. If you have collected $5.0\,cm^3$ of a gas and measured the volume with a syringe that has graduations every $1\,cm^3$, your uncertainty is $\pm 0.5\,cm^3$. This makes the percentage error:

  $$\text{percentage error} = \frac{0.5}{5.0} \times 100 = 10\%$$

- **Validity** refers to both individual measurements and to the whole procedure. If you have a **valid result**, then you know that you measured what you set out to measure. If you have a **valid investigation** then you have measured what you intended to measure and you can be confident that changing the independent variable leads to changes in the dependent variable.

- When you make a conclusion about an investigation then you can make a judgement about the extent to which the evidence collected supports that conclusion. In doing so you are expressing **confidence** in your conclusion. If asked to comment on the confidence in a conclusion then you should consider the following:
  - the limitations in the procedure
  - any uncontrolled variables
  - the effects of errors (systematic and random) on the results
  - the repeatability of the results
  - the precision of the data collected
  - the accuracy of the results

Give some positive aspects of the investigation first, followed by some criticisms. You should refer to specific aspects of the procedure and results, rather than using vague comments such as 'my conclusion is valid because my results are precise and accurate' — this is meaningless without supporting information. For example, you can say that your results are precise because the replicates are close together and there are no anomalous data. Your results may be accurate because they all agree with an expected trend.

Always quote some examples of your raw or processed data in support of your arguments. You can also comment on the resolution of your apparatus, for example by saying that you have measured the dependent variable to a high degree of resolution (e.g. weighing to $0.01\,g$). Resolution refers to the smallest change in the quantity being measured that an instrument can detect (page 8). If you measure $0.2\,g$ of a chemical on a balance that measures to the nearest $0.1\,g$, the balance will not detect a change in mass to $0.19\,g$ or $0.23\,g$ due to the resolution of the equipment.

# ■Required practical activities

## Required practical 1

### Factors affecting the rate of enzyme-controlled reactions

## Background information

This practical requires you to investigate the effect of one variable on the rate of an enzyme-controlled reaction. You will have studied the induced-fit model of enzyme action and the properties of enzymes relating to their tertiary structure. The factors that affect the rate of an enzyme-controlled reaction are:

- enzyme concentration
- substrate concentration
- concentration of competitive and non-competitive inhibitors
- pH
- temperature

The investigation that you carry out will depend on the apparatus and chemicals available, but the most common variables to investigate are pH and temperature.

The enzymes below are popular choices in schools and colleges:

- **Amylase** — hydrolyses starch to maltose and the end-point of the reaction can be clearly visualised using iodine in potassium iodide solution. The end-point is when the blue-black colour no longer appears.
- **Catalase** — catalyses the breakdown of hydrogen peroxide into water and oxygen. The oxygen can be collected and the rate of reaction determined by measuring the volume of gas produced in a specific period of time or the time taken to collect a specific volume of gas. Figure 1 shows some of the different methods that can be used to collect gas.
- **Protease**, for example trypsin — hydrolyses insoluble protein to small, soluble peptides. The time taken for a cloudy protein solution to clear can be measured.

## Guidance through the practical

As with any investigation, it is essential to identify the independent, dependent and control variables.

The **independent variable** will be one of the five factors that affect the rate of an enzyme-controlled reaction. You may be provided with specific values to use — for example, you may be told to use pH 4, 5, 6, 7 and 8 — or you may have to decide suitable values for yourself based on your knowledge of enzyme action.

The **dependent variable** will be a measurement of the time taken for the reaction to complete. This will either be the time taken for the **substrate** to be used up, or the time taken for the **product** to form.

The **control variables** are the ones that need to remain constant. You should be able to state how and why you controlled these variables because identification of control variables is one of the practical skills that will be assessed in the written papers. If your independent variable is temperature, you need to control all of the other factors that could affect the rate of reaction, for example pH using a buffer solution.

**Exam tip**

Always refer to 'iodine in potassium iodide solution' or 'iodine *solution*', never just 'iodine', because iodine is a solid.

**Exam tip**

A question on practical work may include the use of reagents to identify biological molecules. Biuret reagent is used to test for protein. If no protein is present, the solution remains blue. If protein is present, the solution turns purple.

**Exam tip**

Always refer to 'volume' rather than 'amount' of oxygen produced. The word 'amount' is ambiguous and is often wrongly used when volume, concentration or number is the correct term to use.

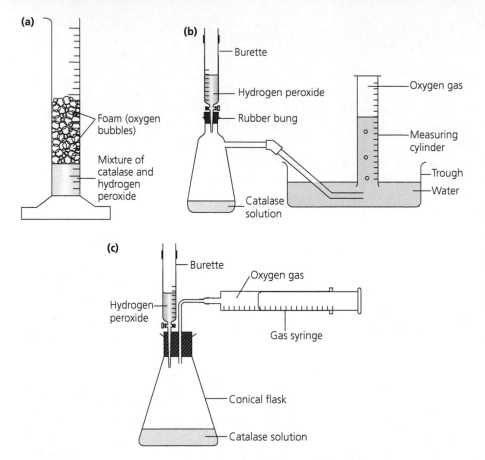

**Figure 1** Different techniques for measuring oxygen production with catalase

The written papers may assess your ability to consider margins of error, accuracy and precision of data. All measurements that you make have some **uncertainty** so measurements are often written with the uncertainty. For example, when temperature is measured the scale usually has intervals of 1°C, so the uncertainty is half of this interval (0.5°C) and so a measurement would be written as, for example, 20.0 ± 0.5°C.

You should consider the uncertainty of the measurements you need to make when selecting suitable apparatus and instrumentation (ATa and ATb). If you need to measure 1 cm³ of solution, a piece of equipment with intervals of 0.1 cm³ will give a smaller uncertainty (±0.05 cm³) than a piece of equipment with intervals of 0.5 cm³ (±0.25 cm³).

## Presentation of results from the practical

Before starting the practical, you should draw a suitable table in which to record your measurements. When drawing a results table, follow the rules given in the practical advice section (page 10). Figure 2 shows an example of a student's results table from an investigation in which the student compared the activity of amylase from two sources.

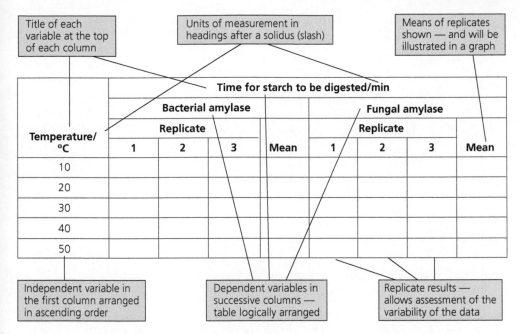

Title of each variable at the top of each column

Units of measurement in headings after a solidus (slash)

Means of replicates shown — and will be illustrated in a graph

| Temperature/ °C | Time for starch to be digested/min | | | | | | | |
| | Bacterial amylase | | | | Fungal amylase | | | |
| | Replicate | | | | Replicate | | | |
| | 1 | 2 | 3 | Mean | 1 | 2 | 3 | Mean |
| 10 | | | | | | | | |
| 20 | | | | | | | | |
| 30 | | | | | | | | |
| 40 | | | | | | | | |
| 50 | | | | | | | | |

Independent variable in the first column arranged in ascending order

Dependent variables in successive columns — table logically arranged

Replicate results — allows assessment of the variability of the data

**Figure 2** A table showing the effect of temperature on starch digestion, with guidance on table structure

The data you collect for the dependent variable will be a measurement of the time taken for the reaction to reach completion. The investigation requires you to determine the **rate** of the reaction, so you will need to process these data. The rate is the speed of the reaction, so it will be per unit time, for example per second ($s^{-1}$) or per minute ($min^{-1}$). If you have found the volume of oxygen produced in a specified time, you would determine the rate using volume/time. You need to include suitable units for rate, so if you collected $10\,cm^3$ of oxygen in 5 minutes, the rate of reaction would be $2\,cm^3$ per minute, expressed as $cm^3\,min^{-1}$.

In other investigations, you may just have a measurement of time. To express this as a rate, you need to calculate the reciprocal of the time, which is 1/time. Again, you need to include the unit — $s^{-1}$, $min^{-1}$ or $h^{-1}$, depending on the measurements taken.

Once you have processed your data, you should present them as a graph. If you have investigated a continuous variable (temperature, pH, enzyme concentration or substrate concentration) your results should be presented as a line graph. If you have investigated the effect of an inhibitor — for example, rate of reaction *with* an inhibitor and rate of reaction *without* an inhibitor — then a bar chart would be appropriate. Your ability to present data graphically will be assessed by examiners in the written papers and also by your teacher as part of the practical endorsement (CPAC 4).

The following rules should be followed when plotting your graph:

■ The independent variable (the factor changed) is on the *x*-axis. The dependent variable (the rate of reaction) is on the *y*-axis.

■ Both axes are fully labelled and have correct units.

■ An appropriate scale has been chosen for each axis.

■ Points have been plotted accurately using saltire crosses (×) so they can be seen clearly.

■ Each point has been joined with a straight line.

**Exam tip**

Use the term **mean** rather than average. Average refers to a central value, which could be the mean, median or mode.

**Exam tip**

When calculating the reciprocal, you could also use 100/time or even 1000/time so that you do not get a rate with too many decimal places.

**Exam tip**

Always choose a scale that is easy to work with, for example multiples of 2, 5 or 10. Avoid using scales that are difficult to work with, such as intervals of 3.

Figure 3 shows a graph that has been plotted following these five rules, whereas the graph shown in Figure 4 does not have a suitable *x*-axis scale and the line has been extrapolated.

**Exam tip**

Always join points with a straight ruled line if you cannot be certain of the intermediate values.

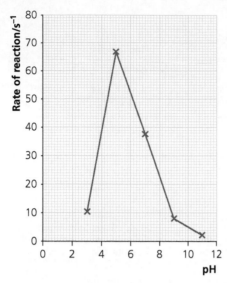

**Figure 3** A graph to show the effect of pH on the activity of amylase. The graph has the axes the correct way round, a suitable scale, clearly labelled axes and correctly plotted points joined with straight lines

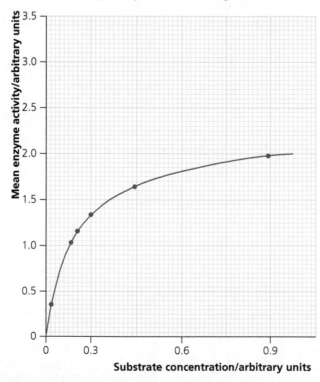

**Figure 4** A graph to show the effect of substrate concentration on urease activity. The graph has a poor choice of *x*-axis scale that is non-linear (does not increase in equal increments)

# Analysis/evaluation of the results

Once you have plotted your graph, you need to use your knowledge of enzyme action to explain your results. You should describe the trend or overall pattern of your results using terms such as increase/decrease, plateau/level off, maximum and directly proportional.

Figure 5 shows some of the common trends seen in graphs, together with descriptions of the trends.

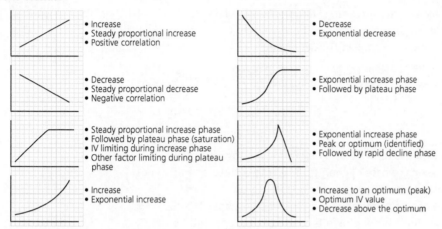

**Figure 5** Graphs showing some common trends and descriptive terms

When you are explaining the shape of a graph, you may find it helpful to number the main sections of your graph and then describe each section.

The graph shown in Figure 6 has three main sections, labelled A, B and C.

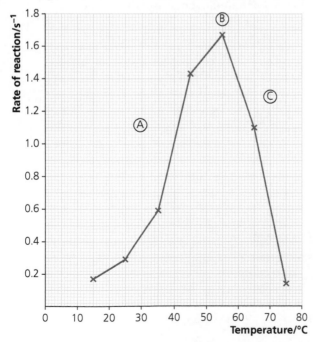

**Figure 6** Graph to show the effect of temperature on the rate of an enzyme-controlled reaction

# Skills Guidance

Section A of the graph shows the rate of reaction increasing between 15°C and 55°C. You should explain this by referring to the increased temperature and its effect on the kinetic energy of the molecules, the number of successful collisions and the formation of enzyme–substrate complexes.

The maximum rate of reaction is reached at 55°C (labelled B). Include the term 'optimum temperature' when you explain this section.

Section C shows the rate decreasing at temperatures above 55°C. Explain this by describing the effect of high temperatures on hydrogen bonds and how this affects the tertiary structure of the enzyme and the shape of the active site.

### Exam tip

You cannot conclude that you have found the optimum temperature for the enzyme if you have not taken measurements of the intermediate values.

## Focus on maths skills

### Calculating the rate of an enzyme-controlled reaction using a tangent to a curve

You may be assessed on your ability to draw and use the slope (gradient) of a tangent to a curve as a measure of rate of change. The role of catalase in the decomposition of hydrogen peroxide was described in the background information section. The rate of this reaction can be found by measuring the volume of oxygen produced per unit time. The initial rate of reaction will be rapid because there are a lot of substrate molecules present and very little product. As the reaction proceeds, there will be fewer substrate molecules available and the rate of reaction will slow down. The initial rate of the reaction can be found using the following method:

1  Select the point at which you want to measure the gradient.
2  Draw a tangent to the curve at your chosen point. (A tangent is a straight line that just touches a curve, but does not cut across it.)
3  From your graph, find the change in the y-axis value and the change in the x-axis value.
4  Calculate the gradient using change in y divided by change in x.

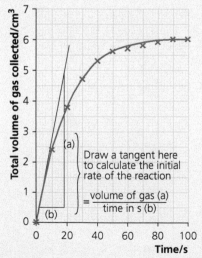

**Figure 7** Calculating the initial rate of an enzyme-controlled reaction using a tangent to a curve

From Figure 7, the change in the $y$-axis value = 4.9 – 0.5 = 4.4 cm$^3$.

The change in the $x$-axis value = 18 – 2 = 16 s.

So the gradient = 4.4/16 = 0.275 cm$^3$ s$^{-1}$.

This method is useful when investigating the rate of an enzyme-controlled reaction as it allows you to measure the change in rate as the reaction progresses.

# Required practical 2

**Preparing and observing a root tip squash**

## Background information

Eukaryotic cells that are able to divide show a cycle of cell growth and division called the **cell cycle**. **Interphase** takes up most of the cell cycle and is when DNA replication occurs. Interphase is followed by **mitosis**, when the cell divides to produce two identical daughter cells. Mitosis can be divided into four main stages:

1 prophase
2 metaphase
3 anaphase
4 telophase

For each of these stages, you should be able to describe the behaviour of the chromosomes and explain the appearance of cells. You could copy and complete Table 2 and then use your textbook to prepare a summary before you complete the practical.

**Exam tip**

Make sure that you can identify the stages of the cell cycle from both diagrams and photographs.

**Table 2** A table that could be used to record the appearance of root tip cells

| Stage of the cell cycle | Description of the cells' appearance | Explanation of the cells' appearance |
|---|---|---|
| Interphase | | |
| Prophase | | |
| Metaphase | | |
| Anaphase | | |
| Telophase | | |

## Guidance through the practical

This practical requires you to complete three activities:

1 Prepare a slide — the tip of a plant root needs to be mounted on a slide, stained so that the chromosomes can be seen clearly, and squashed to produce a single layer of cells.

2 Use an optical microscope — you need to focus the microscope at a suitable magnification to allow individual cells to be seen and counted.

3 Calculate a mitotic index — both the number of cells undergoing mitosis and the total number of cells should be counted. The mitotic index is then calculated using the formula:

$$\text{mitotic index} = \frac{\text{number of cells undergoing mitosis}}{\text{total number of cells}}$$

## *Preparing the slide*

To prepare the slide, you need access to plant roots — onion and garlic are commonly used in schools and colleges. The bulb can be stood on a beaker or conical flask full of water and the roots will be clearly visible after 2–5 days, as shown in Figure 8.

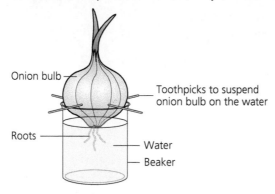

Onion bulb

Toothpicks to suspend onion bulb on the water

Roots

Water

Beaker

**Figure 8** Onion suspended above water

It is important that you only use the very tip of the root, cutting approximately 1 mm off the end, because the **meristematic cells** found here are actively dividing. They should appear small and square when you look at them down the microscope, and the nucleus should be in the centre of the cell (Figure 9). The cells further away from the tip are no longer dividing; they are elongating. These cells will appear longer and the nucleus will not be central.

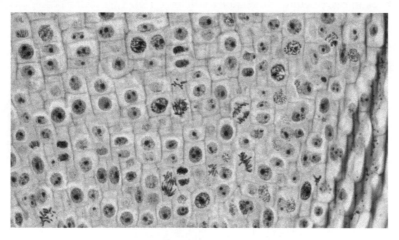

**Figure 9** Meristematic cells from a root tip as seen using an optical microscope at medium power

Once the root tip has been removed, cell division must be halted immediately and the root tip prepared so that it can be observed using an optical microscope. The technique you use will depend on the availability of chemicals and a risk assessment carried out by the school or college, but the main steps are as follows:

1  **Fixing** — this kills the cells while causing minimum changes to them. Place the tissue in ethanoic alcohol and in concentrated hydrochloric acid. This stops cell division and also hydrolyses the middle lamella so that the cells can be separated easily.

The middle lamella is a layer of pectin that cements adjacent plant cells together.

2  **Staining** — place the root tip on a slide and add a stain that will bind to the chromosomes. This may be **toluidine blue**, which stains chromosomes blue, or **acetic orcein**, which stains chromosomes a purple-red colour.

3  **Preparing a root tip squash** — squash the stained root tip by placing a coverslip on top of the root tip and pressing down gently but firmly in the centre of the coverslip. This produces a single layer of cells, so you can see individual cells when you view the slide using a microscope, and allows the transmission of light through the specimen on the slide. Take care when doing this as the coverslip is made of glass and will break easily. Do not let the coverslip move from side to side, as this may damage or break the chromosomes.

## Using an optical microscope

An optical microscope is also known as a light microscope because it relies on the transmission of light through the specimen on the stage. The microscopes used in schools and colleges vary, but they all have the same general structure shown in Figure 10.

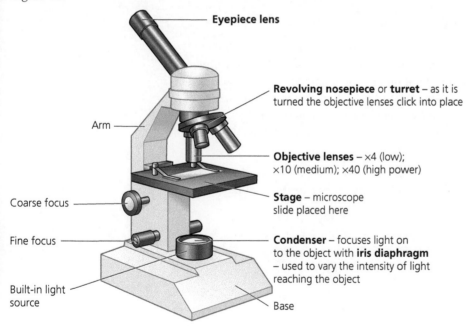

**Figure 10** A typical optical microscope

When using a microscope, you should follow these steps:

1  Carry the microscope with one hand on the arm and the other under the base, and place the microscope on a stable surface in a well-lit area.

2  Turn on the light. You may need to plug the microscope in, or it may have a built-in battery.

3  Select the smallest **objective lens** by turning the turret until you feel the lens 'click' into place.

4  Place your slide on the **stage** and gently slide it under the clips, or into the slide holder if your microscope has a mechanical stage.

5  Looking at the stage from the side, use the **coarse focus** to either raise the stage or lower the lens (depending on the microscope) so that your slide is almost touching the objective lens.

6  Look through the **eyepiece lens**. The circular area that you can see is called the **field of view**.

7  Slowly adjust the coarse focus so that the slide is moving away from the objective lens.

8  Use the **fine focus** to bring the specimen into clear focus.

9  Turn the turret so that the medium objective lens clicks into place. Increasing the magnification decreases the field of view and fewer cells will be visible.

10 Look through the eyepiece lens and slowly adjust the **fine focus** until you can see the specimen clearly. Use a higher magnification if necessary. You are looking for small square cells arranged in rows, as seen in Figure 9.

| Practical tip |
| --- |

If you cannot see a clear image using the medium- or high-power objective lenses, select a lower-power (smaller) lens and refocus at the lower power.

## Calculating a mitotic index

Once you have a clearly focused specimen, you should count the total number of cells that you can see. Record this number in your lab book with a clear description of what the number is — for example, total number of onion root tip cells seen at a magnification of ×100. You should then count the number of cells that are in any of the stages of mitosis (prophase, metaphase, anaphase or telophase) and record this number clearly in your lab book. Table 3 shows an example of a suitable table for recording your results.

Depending on the amount of time available, you could repeat these counts for several fields of view. Divide the number of cells undergoing mitosis by the total number of cells to calculate the mitotic index.

Table 3 An example of a table for recording your results and calculating mitotic index

| Field of view | Total number of cells | Number of cells in stages of mitosis | Mitotic index |
| --- | --- | --- | --- |
| 1 | | | |
| 2 | | | |
| 3 | | | |

# Presentation of results from the practical

Your teacher may ask you to make cell drawings of your specimen in your lab book. Following the guidance on biological drawing on page 35, draw the cells to show the structures you can see at each stage of the cell cycle. Figure 11 shows both good and bad examples of biological drawings. Remember to label your drawing and include the magnification next to it. The maths skills box explains how to use an eyepiece graticule and calculate the magnification.

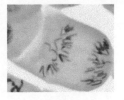

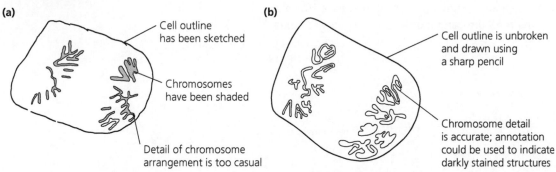

**(a)**
Cell outline
has been sketched

Chromosomes
have been shaded

Detail of chromosome
arrangement is too casual

**(b)**
Cell outline is unbroken
and drawn using
a sharp pencil

Chromosome detail
is accurate; annotation
could be used to indicate
darkly stained structures

**Figure 11** Biological drawings of a root tip cell undergoing mitosis: (a) this drawing makes many common mistakes; (b) an example of a clearly drawn cell

## Analysis/evaluation of the results

In the exam, you might be given data about the duration of one cell cycle and the number of cells observed at each stage of mitosis. You could then be expected to calculate the period of time spent at each stage.

For example, in garlic root tissue, one cell cycle takes 8 hours. There are 50 cells and four of them are in metaphase. Calculate how many minutes these cells spend in metaphase.

The first step is to convert hours to minutes: 8 hours = 480 minutes.

The time spent in metaphase is:

$$\frac{4}{50} \times 480 = 38.4 \text{ minutes}$$

---

### Focus on maths skills

#### Using an eyepiece graticule and calculating magnification

An eyepiece graticule is a glass or plastic disc with a scale on it. It is inserted into the eyepiece lens of a microscope and can be used to measure cells or structures. Before it can be used, it needs to be **calibrated** for each magnification (Figure 12).

Calibrating an eyepiece graticule:
1 Place a **stage micrometer** on the stage of a microscope. A stage micrometer is a glass slide with a scale marked at intervals, for example of 0.1 mm (100 μm) and 0.01 mm (10 μm).

→

2 Focus on the scale on the stage micrometer using the low-power objective lens.
3 Align the scales of the eyepiece graticule and the stage micrometer.
4 Count the number of divisions of the eyepiece graticule that are equivalent to 100 micrometres (100 μm) on the stage micrometer.
5 Calculate the length of one eyepiece division. For example, if 100 μm equals five eyepiece divisions, then each division equals 20 μm.
6 Repeat for the medium- and high-power objective lenses.

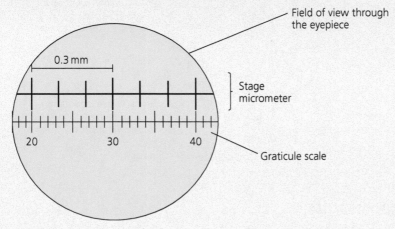

**Figure 12** Calibrating an eyepiece graticule. The eyepiece is aligned with the stage micrometer. 10 divisions on the eyepiece graticule represent 0.3 mm, so each eyepiece graticule division = 0.03 mm or 30 μm

Using an eyepiece graticule to measure objects:
1 Place a prepared slide on the stage of a microscope.
2 Focus on the slide using the low-power objective lens.
3 Use the medium- or high-power objective lens to focus on an individual cell.
4 Measure the length of the cell by counting the number of eyepiece divisions.
5 Work out the **actual length** of the cell in micrometres using your calibrated values.

Calculating the magnification of a drawing:
1 Measure the length of the cell that you have drawn to give the **image length**.
2 Calculate the **magnification** using image length/actual length.
3 This magnification can be written next to your drawing.

# Required practical 3

### Using a calibration curve to estimate water potential

## Background information

There are two elements to this practical — preparing a dilution series and then determining the water potential of plant tissue. Water potential is covered in the 'Transport across cell membranes' section of the specification, where you will have explained osmosis in terms of water potential. Water potential is measured in units of pressure (usually kilopascals, kPa) because it refers to the pressure created by water molecules. Pure water has a water potential of 0 kPa. The addition of any solute to this pure water will lower the water potential and therefore make it negative. Water always moves from higher water potential (less negative) to lower water potential (more negative).

The water potential of plant tissues can be determined by placing them in solutions with known solute concentrations. If the plant tissue *gains* mass, then water has *entered* the tissue by osmosis, and if the tissue *loses* mass, then water has *left* the tissue by osmosis. The concentration at which there is no loss or gain of mass is the one at which there has been no net movement of water by osmosis. This concentration has the same water potential as the plant tissue.

The specification does not name a particular plant tissue that should be used, but many schools and colleges use potatoes because they are readily available, are easy to cut to size, and give results within the time frame of a lesson. The solute is not specified either, but sodium chloride and sucrose are often used.

## Guidance through the practical

### *Preparing a dilution series*

A dilution series is prepared from a stock solution of known concentration, which is then diluted using distilled water. You may be told which concentrations to prepare, or you may have to decide on suitable concentrations for yourself, in which case you should choose even increments that will give you a minimum of 5 or 6 concentrations. For example, with a $1.0 \, mol \, dm^{-3}$ sucrose solution, you could prepare concentrations of 0.2, 0.4, 0.6 and $0.8 \, mol \, dm^{-3}$. Distilled water on its own should also be used to give you a concentration of $0.0 \, mol \, dm^{-3}$.

To prepare the dilution series you need to choose a piece of apparatus with a suitable scale to reduce the uncertainty of your readings. A burette with scale divisions of $0.1 \, cm^3$ would be a more appropriate choice of apparatus than a measuring cylinder with divisions of $0.5 \, cm^3$. The slightly curved surface of a liquid is called the **meniscus**. Take your reading from the bottom of the meniscus, as shown in Figure 13.

Once you have decided on the concentrations that you are going to use, you need to know the volumes of stock solution and distilled water to use. There are two steps to this process:

**Step 1**  Calculate the volume of stock solution. Use the equation:

$$\frac{\text{required concentration}}{\text{concentration of stock solution}} \times \text{final volume required}$$

**Step 2**  Calculate the volume of distilled water to add.

You then subtract the volume calculated in step 1 from the final volume required.

For example, if you wanted to prepare $30 \, cm^3$ of $0.15 \, mol \, dm^{-3}$ sucrose solution from a stock solution of $0.5 \, mol \, dm^{-3}$ sucrose solution:

**Step 1**  $\dfrac{0.15}{0.5} \times 30 = 9 \, cm^3$ stock solution

**Step 2**  $30 - 9 = 21 \, cm^3$ distilled water

Make sure that each solution is poured into a boiling tube or other suitable container that has been clearly labelled with the concentration.

**Exam tip**

Pure water has a water potential of 0 and adding solutes makes it negative.

**Exam tip**

Data should always be recorded to a consistent number of decimal places, so the concentration of the distilled water is recorded as $0.0 \, mol \, dm^{-3}$ rather than just $0 \, mol \, dm^{-3}$.

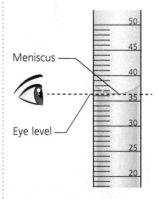

**Figure 13** How to read a volume correctly from the bottom of a meniscus

This type of dilution is called **proportional dilution**. Another type of dilution that you might use is **serial dilution**. This can be carried out using different dilution factors. The method below describes how to dilute by a factor of 10:

1 Add $9\,cm^3$ of dilution liquid (often distilled water) to a series of numbered test tubes.

2 Transfer $1\,cm^3$ of stock solution to tube 1 using a graduated pipette.

3 Mix thoroughly by inverting the test tube. If the stock solution had a concentration of 10% then tube 1 contains a 1% solution as one-tenth of the total volume is stock solution (so 10%/10).

4 Transfer $1\,cm^3$ from tube 1 to tube 2 and mix thoroughly. Tube 2 now contains a 0.1% solution (1%/10).

5 Repeat the transfers until the required dilution series has been produced, as shown in Figure 14.

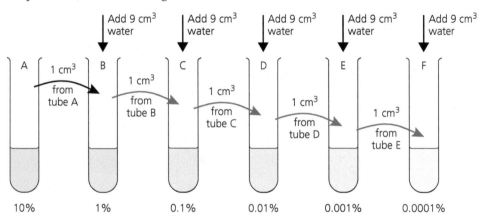

**Figure 14** Making a serial dilution. Each transfer is reducing the concentration of glucose by a factor of 10

Once you have prepared the dilution series, you can move on to the next stage of the practical.

## Determining the water potential of plant tissue

When preparing the plant tissue, it should be handled carefully to prevent damage to the cells. You should devise a method of preparing the plant tissue that ensures a uniform size, shape and surface area. Using a cork borer to produce potato cylinders is a straightforward technique that ensures a consistent diameter and the cylinders can then be cut to the same length. (If using potatoes you should make sure that the 'skin' (corky layer) is removed from the plant tissue.) Alternatively, you may be provided with a knife or a scalpel to cut the plant tissue to an appropriate size. Whether using a cork borer, knife or scalpel, the instrument should be used carefully to minimise the risk of injury (ATj).

The balance that you use to weigh the plant tissue should ideally measure to three decimal places, but two decimal places should give suitable results. The balance should be on a stable surface; most balances have a level indicator and adjustable legs so you can make sure that they are level.

**Practical tip**

Serial dilution can use dilution factors other than 10. To dilute by a factor of 2 you could transfer $5\,cm^3$ each time to produce a total volume of $10\,cm^3$.

**Practical tip**

Use a sharp blade and always cut away from yourself. Cut onto a suitable surface, for example a white tile or wooden board.

Record the mass of each piece of plant tissue as you weigh it, then place it directly into the required concentration and start your stopwatch.

After leaving the pieces of plant tissue in solution for the required period of time, gently blot them dry and weigh them again. You should take your lab book over to the balance with you and record the masses straight into your results table.

As with other investigations, you should identify the control variables and ensure that they remain constant. The significant variables that need controlling include:

- temperature
- source of plant tissue — for example, use the same potato
- size and shape of plant tissue
- batch of stock solution
- length of time the plant tissue is immersed in the solution

For each of these, you should be able to explain how and why you are controlling them.

## Presentation of results from the practical

You should draw your results table in your lab book before starting the practical, ensuring that you have sufficient columns and space for all of the raw data you plan to collect. You can always add columns if necessary, or draw a second table for processed data. A table for **raw data** would need to include columns for:

- the concentration of solute — the units for this may be moles per cubic decimetre $(mol\,dm^{-3})$, which can also be written as molarity (M)
- the initial mass of the plant tissue/g
- the final mass of the plant tissue/g

You will then use your raw data to produce your processed data. Processed data are calculations using your raw data and will include:

- the change in mass/g (final mass minus initial mass)
- the percentage change in mass (see page 29)

You should also convert the concentrations of the sucrose solution to water potential using Table 4.

**Table 4** Conversions of sucrose concentration to water potential

| Concentration of sucrose solution/mol dm$^{-3}$ | Water potential/kPa |
|---|---|
| 0.00 | 0 |
| 0.20 | −540 |
| 0.40 | −1120 |
| 0.60 | −1800 |
| 0.80 | −2580 |
| 1.00 | −3500 |

Your processed data should then be presented as a line graph because the variables are continuous. Figure 15 shows an example of the type of graph you could plot.

The graph should have:

- water potential on the $x$-axis and the percentage change in mass on the $y$-axis
- a $y$-axis scale that allows you to plot both positive and negative values

**Practical tip**

Each piece of plant tissue needs to go into a separate test tube or Petri dish.

**Exam tip**

Remember that the concentration of your solutions refers to the concentration of *solute*, so the solution with the lowest concentration will have the highest water potential.

**Practical tip**

Remember that 1 dm$^3$ equals 1000 cm$^3$.

- a suitable scale, with the same scale divisions on both the positive and negative sections of the y-axis
- points joined with a suitable line

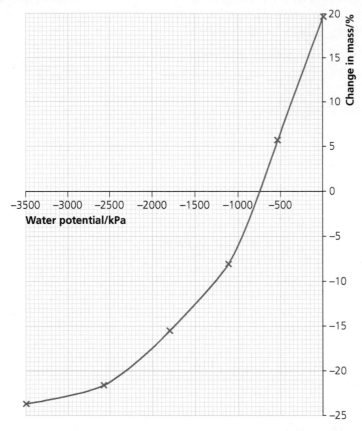

**Figure 15** Graph showing the effect of water potential on the percentage change in mass of plant tissue. The x-axis intercept is equal to the water potential of the plant tissue (−750 kPa)

## Analysis/evaluation of the results

Once you have plotted your graph, you will notice that there are three main sections:

- Above the x-axis where there is an increase in mass.
- The x-axis intercept, where there is no overall change in mass.
- Below the x-axis, where there is a decrease in mass.

For each of these sections, you should be able to explain what is happening to the plant tissue in terms of the loss or gain of water by osmosis, and whether the water potential of the solution is less negative or more negative than the plant tissue.

You can use your graph to determine the water potential of the plant tissue using the x-intercept. Find the point where the line crosses the x-axis and record the water potential. At this point, there is no change in mass and therefore no net movement of water into or out of the plant tissue.

**Exam tip**

Remember that when the solute concentration is *low*, the water potential is *high*, so water enters the cells by osmosis and the plant tissue *gains* mass.

**Referencing**

Remember that all sources should be credited when writing a report in your lab book, to provide evidence for CPAC 5.

If a website is used, you must include the full web address, plus the date and time of access. For example:

> http://www.nuffieldfoundation.org/practical-biology/investigating-
> effect-concentration-blackcurrant-squash-osmosis-chipped-potatoes
> (21/12/2016; 17:15)

If a book is used, you must include the author's name, year of publication, title, edition, city where published and name of publisher. For example:

> Lowrie, P., Smith, M., Bailey, M., Indge, B. and Rowland, M. (2015)
> *AQA A-level Biology 1*, 1st edition, London: Hodder Education.

**Focus on maths skills**

### Percentage change

Calculating percentage change is important because it allows us to compare the change in mass of plant tissue samples that had a different initial mass. It is calculated by:

$$\frac{\text{change in mass}}{\text{initial mass}} \times 100$$

You should include a plus (+) sign to indicate an increase in mass and a minus (−) sign to show a decrease in mass.

You may be assessed on your ability to calculate percentage change, percentage increase and percentage decrease. The principle is always the same:

$$\frac{\text{difference}}{\text{original}} \times 100$$

**Exam tip**

Remember that percentage increase can be greater than 100% because it is possible to have more than a 100% increase. For example, a crop yield that has increased from 80 kg to 190 kg shows a 137.5% increase.

# Required practical 4

**Factors affecting membrane permeability**

## Background information

In this practical, you will investigate the effect of a named variable on the permeability of cell-surface membranes. The cell-surface membrane refers to the plasma membrane that forms the boundary between the cytoplasm and the external environment. Membranes are also found around and in cell organelles, and all have the same basic structure.

The fluid-mosaic structure of cell membranes is covered in the 'Transport across cell membranes' section of the specification, and an important synoptic link to make is between the presence of proteins in membranes and the properties of proteins. Any factor that affects the tertiary structure of a protein, such as temperature or pH, will affect the permeability of the membrane. Similarly, factors that change the fluidity of the phospholipid bilayer of a membrane will affect its permeability. High temperatures and extremes of pH can denature the proteins in cell membranes, leading to an increase in permeability. Some lipid-soluble solvents, such as alcohol, can damage cell membranes, again leading to an increase in permeability.

Any investigation that you carry out will require you to take measurements or make observations about membrane permeability. For that reason, the techniques used generally involve using plant tissues that contain coloured pigments, such as beetroot or red cabbage. Both beetroot and red cabbage contain water-soluble pigments that are in solution in the cell vacuole. When the membranes of these plant tissues are more permeable, the coloured pigment can leak out more readily through the fully permeable cell walls and diffuse into the surrounding solution. Both the cell-surface membrane *and* the **tonoplast** — the membrane around the vacuole (Figure 16) — must be disrupted for the pigment to leave the vacuole. The intensity of the colour of the surrounding solution is directly related to membrane permeability and could be measured **semi-quantitatively** by comparing the solutions to colour standards, or **quantitatively** using a colorimeter.

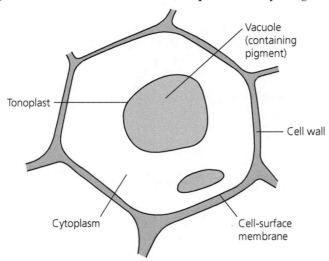

**Figure 16** A plant cell, showing the structures through which pigments must diffuse

## Guidance through the practical

The independent variable investigated is often temperature, because as there is a clear relationship between temperature and membrane permeability there is a good link to the proteins section of the specification. You may also investigate the effect of different types of alcohol or of different concentrations of an alcohol, for example ethanol, on membrane permeability.

The availability of equipment will affect your choice of dependent variable, because a colorimeter is required to obtain quantitative data.

If you investigate the effect of temperature, important variables to control would include:

■ source of plant tissue
■ time in solution
■ size and shape of plant tissue

Any plant tissue that is used must be fresh; preservation techniques, such as pickling or canning, would have damaged the cell membranes. Your method of cutting the plant tissue will depend on the type of plant you use, but with beetroot a cork borer

**Practical tip**

Quantitative results are numerical values, whereas qualitative results are non-numerical or descriptive.

Semi-quantitative results allow you to estimate the amount or concentration of a substance.

can be used to cut out cylinders and then these cylinders can be cut into equal-sized discs. When you cut the plant tissue, particularly if you use beetroot, some pigment will be released so you will need to rinse the discs thoroughly using distilled water. Care should be taken when using cork borers, scalpels and knives.

## Method 1 Semi-quantitative technique

### Part 1

For this method, the first step is preparing a series of colour standards. You will then use these to compare your test solutions against when investigating membrane permeability. You need to start with distilled water and a solution of pure plant extract, for example beetroot extract, and then use these to prepare a series of different concentrations at equal intervals. The distilled water will be 0% and the pure plant extract will be 100%, so your dilutions may be 20%, 40%, 60% and 80%.

Table 5 shows the volumes of water and plant extract that you could use to make 10 cm³ of each concentration of extract.

**Table 5** How to dilute a plant extract using proportional dilution

| Concentration of extract/% | 0 | 20 | 40 | 60 | 80 | 100 |
|---|---|---|---|---|---|---|
| Volume of distilled water/cm³ | 10 | 8 | 6 | 4 | 2 | 0 |
| Volume of plant extract/cm³ | 0 | 2 | 4 | 6 | 8 | 10 |

Once you have a series of colour standards, you can investigate your chosen variable. This example will now focus on temperature.

### Part 2

1   Set up water baths at the required temperatures, for example, 20°C, 30°C, 40°C, 50°C and 60°C. Ideally these will be thermostatically controlled water baths, but if these are not available then a beaker of water can be used. It is important to monitor the temperature throughout the investigation using a thermometer checked at regular intervals. Hot water can be added to the water bath if the temperature starts to fall.

2   Label clean test tubes with each temperature.

3   Measure the same volume of distilled water into each tube.

4   Place the same number of beetroot discs, or other suitable plant tissue, into each tube.

5   Leave the tubes in the water bath for the same period of time.

6   Gently shake the tubes at regular intervals to maintain the diffusion gradient for the pigment.

7   At the end of the time in the water bath, remove the beetroot discs so that no more pigment diffuses out.

8   Compare the colour of the solution from each temperature with your range of colour standards and record the percentage concentration in a suitable results table.

There are two main issues with this method:

■ Matching to the colour standards is subjective.

■ The colour you obtain may not match any of your colour standards.

Subjective results depend on the interpretation or judgement of the person making the observation.

### Method 2 Quantitative technique using a colorimeter

If a colorimeter is available for use, the issues associated with using colour standards do not apply. You can just carry out part 2 of the method described above so that you have test tubes containing coloured solution from each temperature. A colorimeter can be used to measure the absorbance of each solution, and this value can be recorded in your results table.

### Using a colorimeter

A colorimeter is an instrument that can be used to determine the concentration of solute in a solution. It does this by shining light through a solution and measuring either the **transmission** (the percentage of light that passes through the solution) or the **absorbance** (the light absorbed by the solution). The concentration of the solute is proportional to the absorbance of the solution, so a more concentrated solution will have a higher absorbance.

Colorimeters have coloured filters and can be adjusted to select a suitable wavelength of light. You should choose the colour that is complementary to the colour of your solution, as this will give the maximum absorbance. Complementary colours are opposite each other on the colour wheel, as shown in Figure 17, so you should select a green filter if your solution is red.

Some colorimeters require you to use a cuvette (Figure 18), whereas others are designed to accommodate both test tubes and cuvettes.

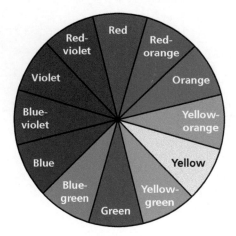

**Figure 17** A colour wheel

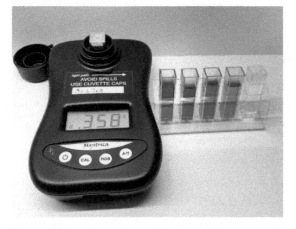

**Figure 18** A colorimeter with a sample in a cuvette

> **Practical tip**
>
> A colorimeter can measure absorbance or percentage transmission.

> A **cuvette** is a clear, straight-sided container made of glass or plastic.

Before taking readings with the colorimeter, you need to set it to give an absorbance reading of zero (or a percentage light transmission of 100%). The solution that you use to do this is called a 'blank' and will be distilled water in this practical. When using a colorimeter, you are looking for a change in colour, so the blank is not always distilled water.

## Presentation of results from the practical

Your results table should be drawn in your lab book before you start the practical. The independent variable, for example temperature, should be in the first column and the dependent variable in the following column. The dependent variable may be your

> **Practical tip**
>
> Absorbance does *not* have units because it is a ratio (of the amount of light that passes through a solution compared with the amount of light that passes into the solution).

*estimation* of pigment concentration if you used colour standards, or your reading of absorbance or light transmission from the colorimeter. Remember to include units in the column headings only.

You should plot a graph of your results with the factor that you changed on the *x*-axis and either the estimated pigment concentration or the absorbance on the *y*-axis. The graph will be a line graph if you have investigated temperature, pH or alcohol concentration, as these are all continuous variables. Remember to join the points with straight lines if you cannot be certain of the intermediate values.

## Analysis/evaluation of the results

In your analysis of your results, you should *describe* any trend or pattern that you can see, using values to illustrate this.

You should then *explain* the pattern or trend using your scientific knowledge. If the absorbance of a solution is *high* (or the percentage light transmission is *low*), a lot of the light entering the solution has been absorbed, meaning that the solution is darker, so in this investigation more pigment has been released. For more pigment to pass into the solution, both the cell-surface membrane *and* the tonoplast must be more permeable. You should explain how the factor you are investigating has increased this permeability.

### Focus on maths skills

#### Linear relationship

You should understand that the equation below represents a linear relationship:

$$y = mx + c$$

where $y$ = the dependent variable, $m$ = the gradient of the line, $x$ = the independent variable and $c$ = the intercept on the *y*-axis.

If $c = 0$, the line goes through the origin, so that $y$ is directly proportional to $x$. This relationship is shown in Figure 19 for the effect of enzyme concentration on the rate of reaction.

You can calculate the rate of change by finding the gradient of the line $\left(\dfrac{dy}{dx}\right)$.

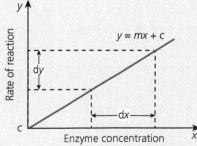

**Figure 19** Graph showing the effect of enzyme concentration on rate of reaction (where substrate is not a limiting factor)

# Required practical 5

### Dissection of an organ or system from an animal or plant

## Background information

The organ or system that you will dissect is not prescribed by AQA, leaving the choice to individual schools and colleges. You could dissect an entire gas exchange system or mass transport system, or you may dissect one organ from within the system, such as a heart.

The specification covers mass transport in both mammals and plants, and gas exchange in insects, fish and dicotyledonous plants. You must be familiar with the features of the mass transport or gas exchange system before you carry out your dissection.

## Guidance through the practical

This practical gives you the opportunity to develop two important skills:

- Safely using instruments for dissection (ATj).
- Producing a scientific drawing with annotations (ATe).

If you are using an animal organ or system, the most important factor is the freshness of the material. Students are often put off dissection because of the smell, but fresh organs will not smell very strong. Remember that any animal material that you use should be kept in a sealed container and stored in the fridge. If you are storing it for more than a day, it can be frozen and then defrosted overnight in the fridge prior to use.

The most common dissections in schools and colleges are hearts or fish heads, as these are cheap and readily available. Hearts can be bought pre-packed from supermarkets but these tend to be 'trimmed', which means that the blood vessels and atria have been removed, whereas a butcher may be able to supply an 'untrimmed' heart. Fish heads are often given away free of charge from fish counters or market stalls.

Other possible dissections are the lungs of a mammal, the gas exchange system of a large insect such as a locust, or a plant mass transport system. The freedom to choose to dissect a plant organ or system makes this practical accessible to all students, including those who prefer not to use animals.

A dissection must be planned and carried out methodically, as its aim is to study the anatomy of the organ or system rather than just hacking it to pieces. You may be given a method to follow or you may be asked to research your own method. Following written instructions is an important skill and provides evidence for CPAC 1.

Preparation is essential and you should ensure that you have all of the equipment you need prior to beginning your dissection.

Both safety and hygiene must be considered, and you may be asked to write a risk assessment before beginning the practical. This should be clearly recorded in your lab book and, together with your teacher's observations of your technique, will provide

> **Exam tip**
>
> Be specific when stating where gas exchange takes place:
> - The gill filaments or gill lamellae, not just the gills.
> - The alveolar epithelium, not just the lungs.
> - The mesophyll, not just the leaves.

evidence for CPAC 3. A risk assessment is often recorded in a table, with hazards, risks and control measures identified. Table 6 shows a student's risk assessment for a heart dissection.

Table 6 Hazards, risks and control measures associated with carrying out a heart dissection

| Hazards | Risks | Control measures |
| --- | --- | --- |
| Scalpel | You might cut yourself | Use a sharp, rust-free blade<br>Cut away from yourself |
| Handling the heart | You might contaminate the work bench<br>There may be bacteria on or in the heart | Wipe down the bench with disinfectant at the end<br>Wash hands thoroughly at the end of the practical |

The following safety precautions should be taken when dissecting an animal organ or system:

- You should wear a disposable plastic apron or lab coat.
- You could wear disposable gloves if they are available.
- Any cuts or open wounds should be covered with waterproof dressings.
- Scalpels and other instruments should be handled with care.
- Materials such as organs and plastic gloves should be disposed of safely.
- All instruments and surfaces should be disinfected at the end of the session.
- Hands should be washed thoroughly with soap and warm water.

## Presentation of results from the practical

This practical provides you with an excellent opportunity to present your results in a different format instead of the tables and graphs that are commonly required. Photographs of your dissection can be stuck directly into your lab book, then labelled and annotated. Alternatively, you could paste the photo into a word document then label and annotate before printing it off and sticking it in your lab book. You can also develop your skills of observation by accurately drawing the structures and tissues that you can see (Figure 20). There are a number of rules to follow with biological drawing:

- Use a sharp pencil.
- Do not shade or use colour.
- Use unbroken lines; do not sketch.
- Label the structures and include brief annotations.
- Include a scale or the magnification.

There are three main types of biological drawing you may complete during the A-level course:

- **Cell drawings** show the components of individual cells as observed using an optical microscope.
- **Tissue maps** show the location of tissues in an organ or organism.
- **Body plans** show the main body parts of a dissected organism.

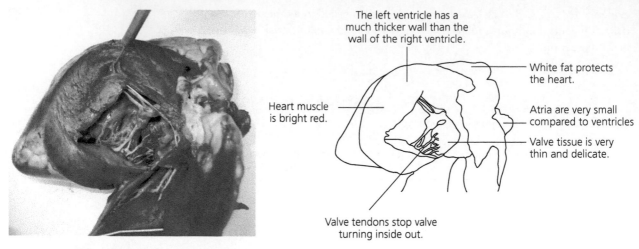

**Figure 20** A photo showing a section of a heart, together with an annotated biological drawing

## Analysis/evaluation of the results

Once you have finished your dissection, you should write a description of the structures that you observed and relate these to your biological knowledge. For example, with a heart dissection you could describe and explain the relative thickness of the chamber walls, the shape of the valves or the strength of the tendons. With a mammalian lung dissection, you could describe and explain the spongy texture of the lungs, the ridged texture of the trachea and bronchi, and differences between the pulmonary artery and pulmonary vein.

# Required practical 6

### Using aseptic techniques to investigate the effect of antimicrobials

## Background information

This practical requires you to investigate the effect of an antimicrobial substance on microbial growth. An antimicrobial substance is any chemical that either kills a microbe or inhibits its growth. Antimicrobials include:

- disinfectants, for example bleach, which can be used on non-living surfaces to kill microbes
- antiseptics, for example ethanol, which are applied to living tissue or skin to reduce the risk of infection
- antibiotics, for example penicillin, which are used to destroy microbes in the body

Microbe is a term that can apply to any microscopic organism, including bacteria, fungi, parasites and viruses.

Antibiotics are a group of chemicals that are used to treat or prevent bacterial infections. There are many different antibiotics with different mechanisms of action — for example, penicillin inhibits cell wall synthesis in growing bacteria.

Testing bacteria for their sensitivity to antibiotics allows doctors to prescribe the correct antibiotic at an effective dosage. This is important in minimising the rise of antibiotic-resistant bacteria.

**Exam tip**

Antibiotic resistance arises from a random mutation that leads to a new allele of a gene. As this new allele is advantageous, it is inherited by the next generation and the frequency of the allele increases in the population.

# Guidance through the practical

This practical gives you the opportunity to use aseptic technique to culture bacteria, and to use a range of apparatus and materials including **agar plates** and **nutrient broth** (ATi).

Agar plates are sterile plastic Petri dishes that have had molten nutrient agar poured into them and are used for culturing bacteria. Nutrient agar is supplied in powder form and is mixed with distilled water and heated before use. The molten agar solidifies as it cools to form a jelly-like substance and microorganisms can grow on the surface. Nutrient agar contains the carbohydrates, organic nitrogen (in the form of peptone — partly digested protein), vitamins and sodium chloride required for the growth of a wide range of microbes, as well as agar powder.

Nutrient broth is a liquid growth medium that contains the nutrients needed for bacterial growth, but does not contain agar. Bacteria can be cultured in small glass bottles containing nutrient broth.

**Aseptic technique** refers to the methods used to prevent contamination by microbes. There are many factors to consider and so your teacher may demonstrate these techniques to you.

- Ensure that the bench or work surface has been thoroughly cleaned and disinfected.
- Light a Bunsen burner and work near the lit Bunsen throughout the practical; the warm air current will create an updraft that reduces the risk of air-borne microbes contaminating your agar.
- Use sterile equipment.

Disposable loops, spreaders and pipettes may be provided in sterile, sealed packages. Alternatively the technician may have sterilised equipment by **autoclaving** (heating at high temperature and pressure).

A Bunsen burner can also be used to sterilise equipment: metal loops can be held in the hottest part of the flame until they glow red hot; glass spreaders can be dipped in ethanol and then passed through the flame to allow the alcohol to burn off.

Remember to let the equipment cool down before it comes into contact with the bacteria, but do not put sterilised equipment down on the bench before use or it may become contaminated.

Your school or college will have chosen the bacteria that you use — they must be easy to culture at low temperatures and should present no risk to health. Common choices include *Bacillus megaterium*, *Escherichia coli* (*E. coli*) and *Micrococcus luteus*.

Before removing a sample of bacteria in broth from the bottle, you may be told to 'flame the neck of the bottle'. This means that you should remove the lid, pass the neck of the bottle through the flame, remove your sample using a sterile pipette, pass the neck of the bottle through the flame again and replace the lid. The bottle does not need to be held in the flame for a long period of time. This process of flaming warms the air around the neck of the bottle so that movement of air is out of the bottle, which prevents contamination of the broth by microbes in the air.

When adding the bacteria to your agar plate, the lid of the Petri dish should be lifted as little as possible. You should then use a sterile spreader to give an even covering

**Practical tip**

Nutrient agar is just one of the many types of agar used for culturing microorganisms. Agar, which is extracted from algae, can be added to different liquid growth media to produce selective, indicator or enriched agar plates.

**Practical tip**

Care must be taken if using ethanol near an open flame because it is flammable.

**Practical tip**

Note that the names of the bacteria are binomials and represent the genus and the species. The genus begins with an upper-case letter, and the species with a lower-case letter. In print, the names are *italicised*, but when handwritten in your lab books, they should be underlined.

over the surface of the agar. After incubation, this will give a continuous layer of bacteria called a **bacterial lawn**.

You should use sterile forceps to place your antimicrobial agent on the agar plate, again lifting the lid as little as possible. You might use a multidisc, which is a ring with different antimicrobial agents, or individual paper discs impregnated with antibiotics. Alternatively, you could make your own paper discs using sterile filter paper soaked in different concentrations of bleach.

The lid of the Petri dish should be held in place with two pieces of tape. It should not be sealed all the way around as this may favour the growth of potentially harmful anaerobic bacteria. The plate should be incubated upside down in an incubator at no more than 25°C. Inverting the plates during incubation means that condensation drips onto the lid rather than on the surface of the agar. Keeping the temperature of the incubator well below human body temperature reduces the risk of growing microbes that are pathogenic to humans.

Incubate the plate for 48 hours then, *without removing the lid* of the Petri dish, examine the growth of the bacteria. You should see clear zones around one or more of the discs where bacterial growth has been inhibited. These clear zones are called **zones of inhibition** (Figure 21). The larger the zone, the more effective the antimicrobial. The radius of each clear zone should be measured and recorded in a suitable results table.

Figure 22 shows the effect of eight antibiotics in a multidisc (mast ring) on the growth of bacteria. Different antibiotics are contained in the arms of the mast ring, so that sensitivity to many antibiotics can be tested simultaneously.

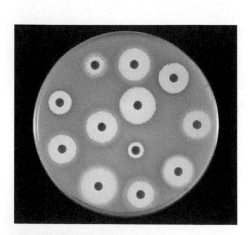

**Figure 21** Photograph showing bacteria growing on an agar plate, with zones of inhibition of varying diameters around the antibiotic discs

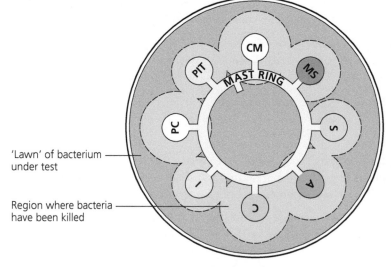

'Lawn' of bacterium under test

Region where bacteria have been killed

**Figure 22** Diagram showing how a multidisc (or mast ring) with different antibiotics affects bacterial growth. The 'clear' areas are zones of inhibition of varying sizes

It is important to disinfect the benches and dispose of agar plates safely at the end of the practical session. Hands should be washed thoroughly with soap and warm water after handling microbes.

## Presentation of results from the practical

You could take a photograph of your plate and stick it in your lab book, or you could draw a diagram of your plate, ensuring that it is an accurate record of your observations.

A table should be drawn with the name of each antibiotic in the first column and the radius of each zone of inhibition in the next column. As each zone of inhibition may not be uniform, you should take several readings and calculate a mean. Measurements should be recorded in millimetres, and you should take each measurement from the centre of the disc. It may be easier to determine the mean diameter and then use this to calculate the radius.

You can add a further column for processed data and use the mean radius to calculate the area of the zone of inhibition for each antibiotic. Remember to include suitable units for area in the column heading (probably mm$^2$).

You could display your results graphically:

- If you have used different antibiotics, you should draw a bar chart with the type of antibiotic on the $x$-axis and the area of the zone of inhibition on the $y$-axis. The bars should not be touching each other, as different antibiotics are an example of categorical data.
- You may have used **serial dilution** to prepare different concentrations of one antimicrobial. In this case you should draw a line graph, as concentration is an example of continuous data, with concentration on the $x$-axis and area of the zone of inhibition on the $y$-axis.

## Analysis/evaluation of the results

You should explain your observations and measurements using your scientific knowledge, and may have to use different sources to research the antibiotics and microbe that you used. If you have used different antibiotics there may be zones of inhibition around some of the discs but not around others, so your analysis should suggest why this occurred. Antibiotics have different mechanisms of action, so may not be effective against the microbe that you used. Alternatively, the lack of a zone of inhibition could indicate antibiotic resistance. You could also consider the physical properties of the antibiotic in terms of the size of the molecules and how this affects their rate of diffusion through the agar.

# Required practical 7

### Using chromatography to investigate leaf pigments

## Background information

The leaves of plants contain photosynthetic pigments that absorb light energy and transfer it to chemical energy in the molecules formed during photosynthesis. These photosynthetic pigments are found in the chloroplasts of eukaryotic cells, embedded in their thylakoid membranes.

**Exam tip**

You may be tested on your ability to calculate the area of a circle using $\pi r^2$ and the circumference of a circle using $2\pi r$, where $r$ = radius and $\pi$ = 3.14.

Categorical data relate to category, such as qualitative data, as opposed to numerical data — for example, names of bacteria or types of antibiotic.

There are many different pigments found in plants, but they all reflect certain wavelengths of light, making them appear coloured — for example, chlorophyll reflects green light. Leaves can contain different pigments, including:

- chlorophyll a — a blue-green pigment that absorbs violet/blue and red light
- chlorophyll b — a yellow-green pigment that absorbs blue and orange/red light
- carotenoids — yellow or yellow-orange pigments that absorb violet, blue and green light
- anthocyanins — red, purple or blue pigments that are not involved in photosynthesis

The carotenoids, including carotene and xanthophyll, are known as accessory pigments and absorb wavelengths of light that chlorophyll cannot.

Paper chromatography can be used to separate a mixture of molecules, for example a mixture of plant pigments. A solvent called the **extraction solvent** is used to extract pigments from a leaf and then a **running solvent** is used to draw the pigments up a piece of filter paper. As the running solvent travels up the filter paper, the pigment molecules are carried up the paper in solution. The rate at which they are carried depends on the solubility of the pigments, the size of the pigment molecules, and the affinity of the pigments for the filter paper (their tendency to adhere or 'stick' to the filter paper).

The filter paper should be left in the solvent for long enough for the pigments to be separated and until the solvent almost reaches the top of the filter paper.

## Guidance through the practical

This practical gives you the opportunity to use paper chromatography (AT g), and the full title of the practical specifies that you should investigate leaves from different plants. One of the suggestions is that you compare leaves from shade-tolerant and shade-intolerant plants. Shade-tolerant plants are those that are able to photosynthesise at low light intensities, such as the European beech, whereas shade-intolerant plants like the silver birch need very high light intensities.

In a woodland, most of the red and blue light is absorbed by the shade-intolerant canopy plants, but far-red light (about 730 nm) and green light can penetrate the canopy. Shade-tolerant plants need photosynthetic pigments that allow them to maximise the absorption of light of these wavelengths.

You could also compare leaves that are different colours. Some leaves appear different colours throughout the year, like those of *Begonia*, which are red, and *Oxalis*, which are purple, or leaves could be collected in the autumn and the pigments present compared.

Figure 23 shows one way that paper chromatography could be set-up.

The first step in this practical is to set up boiling tubes containing a small volume of the running solvent that you are using and seal them with bungs. This will allow the air inside the tubes to become saturated with the solvent.

You should then collect a strip of filter or chromatography paper and draw a *pencil* line called the **origin** about 2 cm from the bottom. You must use pencil as ink may be soluble in the solvent that you use. The chromatography paper should be narrow

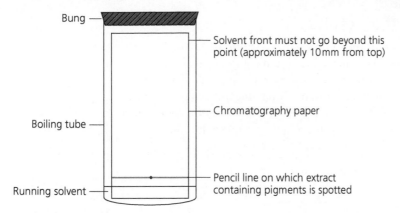

**Figure 23** Diagram showing how to set up paper chromatography

enough not to touch the sides of the boiling tube as this may cause the solvent front to travel at an angle.

The next step is extracting the pigments. This can be achieved by grinding the leaf with a small amount of extraction solvent, such as propanone, using a mortar and pestle. A capillary tube can be used to spot the pigment extract onto the origin line. This is most effective if the paper is allowed to dry between applications to build up a concentrated spot of pigment. Alternatively, the pigments can be transferred directly from the leaf onto the filter paper by placing a leaf disc on the origin line and firmly crushing it with a glass rod.

You should then place the chromatography paper in the boiling tube, making sure that the end of the paper touches the solvent, but that the solvent is below the origin line. If the solvent is above the origin, the pigment will just be 'washed off' the paper. The bung should be replaced and the boiling tube left in a boiling tube rack.

The solvent will gradually rise up the paper and should be left until it *almost* reaches the top. You then need to remove the paper from the solvent and use a pencil to immediately draw a line to mark how far the solvent has travelled. This line is called the **solvent front**. You should do this immediately because you will not be able to see the solvent front once the chromatography paper has dried.

Your chromatography paper with the pigment spots is called a **chromatogram**.

## Presentation of results from the practical

Your chromatogram should be left to dry and then can be stuck in your lab book. Use a pencil to draw around each pigment spot, as they may fade with time. You should also number each pigment to make it easier to refer to in your analysis.

Draw a results table for each chromatogram, with the number allocated to the pigment spots in the first column, their colour in the second column and the distance from the origin to the centre of the pigment spot recorded in mm in the final column.

Process your data by calculating the Rf value for each pigment using this formula:

$$Rf\,value = \frac{distance\ from\ the\ origin\ to\ the\ centre\ of\ the\ pigment\ spot}{distance\ from\ the\ origin\ to\ the\ solvent\ front}$$

These Rf values can be recorded in an additional column in your results table.

## Analysis/evaluation of the results

The Rf value is a ratio of the distance travelled by the pigment and the distance travelled by the solvent. Calculating this value allows you to compare results with others because the ratio for a pigment will be the same even if the actual distances are different. You could identify the pigments on your chromatogram by researching the expected Rf values for each pigment. If there are differences between your values and the expected values, you could suggest possible reasons for these differences.

You should have chromatograms for at least two different leaves and should carry out some research to explain why the leaves contain different pigments.

# Required practical 8

### Factors affecting dehydrogenase activity in chloroplasts

## Background information

In this practical, you are measuring the rate of the **Hill reaction** in isolated chloroplasts. Robert Hill carried out this investigation in 1938 and concluded that water had been split into hydrogen and oxygen.

Before beginning this practical, you need a clear understanding of both the light-dependent and the light-independent reactions of photosynthesis. The light-dependent reaction involves chlorophyll molecules, which are located in the thylakoid membranes, absorbing light energy and losing electrons in a process called **photoionisation**. The electrons are taken up by an electron carrier and then passed along a series of carriers in an electron transfer chain. The electrons lose energy as they pass along the chain to each carrier, and some of this energy is used to synthesise ATP.

Light energy is also used to split a molecule of water in a process known as **photolysis**. This produces protons, electrons and oxygen. Protons and electrons are taken up by an electron carrier called NADP, therefore **reducing** the NADP. The oxygen is used in respiration or diffuses out of the leaf through the stomata.

In summary, the light-dependent reaction produces ATP and reduced NADP, together with oxygen (from the photolysis of water). The ATP and reduced NADP are used in the light-independent reaction of photosynthesis.

DCPIP (2,6-dichlorophenol-indophenol) is a blue dye that acts as an electron acceptor. DCPIP is blue when **oxidised**, and accepting electrons **reduces** the DCPIP, causing it to decolourise. If DCPIP is added to a suspension of isolated chloroplasts, the DCPIP accepts electrons from the electron transfer chain. This reduces the DCPIP, so it changes colour from blue to colourless.

## Guidance through the practical

This practical requires you to investigate the effect of a factor on the activity of chloroplasts. The thylakoids in chloroplasts contain pigments that absorb light, and proteins that are involved in the transfer of electrons. These proteins form the electron transfer chain, which consists of a number of electron carriers embedded in

**Exam tip**

NAD**P** is an electron carrier in **p**hotosynthesis. Do not mix this up with NAD, which is involved in respiration.

**Exam tip**

Remember **OIL RIG**:

**O**xidation **i**s **l**oss of electrons or hydrogen (or gain of oxygen).

**R**eduction **i**s **g**ain of electrons or hydrogen (or loss of oxygen).

the thylakoid membranes. You can investigate any factors that affect the pigments, or any that influence the components of the electron transfer chain.

During this practical, you will choose one factor as your independent variable and ensure that the other factors are controlled.

You can investigate the effect of light intensity and light wavelength on the rate of photosynthesis using the Hill reaction. Some weedkillers act on chloroplasts by inhibiting components of the electron transfer chain and therefore preventing the production of ATP and reduced NADP. Ammonium hydroxide has a similar effect and could be used to investigate the effect of these weedkillers on the rate of photosynthesis.

The effect of light intensity could be investigated by placing your reaction tube at different distances from a lamp. The effect of different wavelengths of light could be investigated by placing filters of different colours (e.g. blue, green and red) between the lamp and the reaction tubes, or wrapping the tubes in the different filters.

Weedkillers could be investigated using ammonium hydroxide to mimic their effects. In theory, the effect of different weedkillers could be investigated, or the effect of a weedkiller at different concentrations. However, a full risk assessment would be necessary to determine whether weedkillers could be safely used in the laboratory.

A source of chloroplasts needs to be selected and the plant material prepared. Spinach leaves are a good choice as they are readily available. These should be prepared by removing the stalks and midribs, which are too tough to blend and may not contain many chloroplasts.

You will need to isolate chloroplasts from the plant material by blending the leaves with ice-cold buffer solution and then filtering the solution. The blending breaks open the cell walls, releasing the cell contents, and filtering removes the cell walls and other debris to leave a suspension of chloroplasts. The buffer needs to be ice-cold to slow down enzyme activity and reduce damage to the chloroplasts. The buffer should also have the same water potential as the cytoplasm so that there is no net movement of water into or out of the chloroplasts by osmosis.

A small volume of your chloroplast suspension can be measured into a test tube and DCPIP added. You can then measure the time taken for the DCPIP to decolourise in different conditions, depending on the independent variable that you chose.

Variables that you will need to control include:
- source of chloroplasts — use the same suspension throughout your investigation
- volume of chloroplast suspension
- volume of DCPIP
- concentration of DCPIP

You will need to ensure consistency when determining the end-point of the reaction and should prepare a colour standard to determine when the DCPIP has completely decolourised. This will be a tube containing just chloroplast suspension and water (use the same volume of water as DCPIP).

**Practical tip**

If the colour change takes more than 2–3 minutes the DCPIP can be diluted.

## Presentation of results from the practical

All results should be recorded in a suitable table with full column headings and units in the column headings only. When recording time, you should never have mixed units, for example, minutes and seconds. Convert the minutes into seconds and consider whether it is appropriate to include hundredths of a second.

As you have measured the time taken for DCPIP to decolourise, you can calculate the rate using 1/time, with a unit of $s^{-1}$.

Plot a graph of your results with the factor that you investigated, such as light intensity or concentration of ammonium hydroxide, on the $x$-axis and rate of photosynthesis on the $y$-axis. These are all continuous data, so your graph will be a line graph. Draw a bar chart if you have used different inhibitors or different filters (if you do not know the wavelength of light that passes through each one).

## Analysis/evaluation of the results

You should describe any patterns or trends shown by your results, and then explain these using your scientific knowledge. Remember that the faster the rate of decolourisation, the higher the rate of the light-dependent stage.

Researching and referencing are important skills that are assessed by your teacher as evidence that you have met CPAC 5. You could take the opportunity to research relevant applications of your findings, such as:

- determining the most effective light intensity for photosynthesis in different plants
- describing the effects of different wavelengths of light on the rate of photosynthesis
- determining the optimum concentration of an inhibitor to use as a weedkiller
- selecting the most effective weedkiller

### Focus on maths skills

#### Recording times

When recording the time taken, you should never include mixed units in a results table, i.e. minutes *and* seconds. Sometimes students record the reading of 6:30 (6 minutes and 30 seconds) from a stopwatch as 6.30 minutes when it should be 6.5 minutes (30 seconds is 0.5 minutes).

You should convert the minutes into seconds, so 6:30 would be recorded as 390 seconds.

# Required practical 9

**Factors affecting the rate of respiration in single-celled organisms**

## Background information

This practical requires knowledge of respiration, but also includes a synoptic link to enzymes, because respiration involves a series of enzyme-controlled reactions. Respiration produces ATP and has four main stages:

- glycolysis
- link reaction
- Krebs cycle
- oxidative phosphorylation

> **Practical tip**
>
> Determining the end-point of a reaction is difficult and subjective. It is unlikely that you could determine the end-point to the nearest second, and definitely not to the nearest hundredth of a second.

> **Practical tip**
>
> Remember that any sources that you use, whether websites, journals or books, should be credited and referenced appropriately.

Glycolysis occurs in the cytoplasm and produces pyruvate, reduced NAD and ATP. The pyruvate is actively transported into the matrix of the mitochondria.

The link reaction occurs in the mitochondrial matrix and uses the pyruvate and coenzyme A to produce acetylcoenzyme A. This process also produces reduced NAD and carbon dioxide.

The Krebs cycle also occurs in the matrix and involves a series of oxidation–reduction reactions that produce reduced NAD, reduced FAD and ATP.

Oxidative phosphorylation takes place in the mitochondria using proteins, such as carriers and enzymes, embedded in the inner mitochondrial membrane. Electrons from reduced NAD and reduced FAD are transferred down the electron transfer chain (a series of electron carriers) and the energy released is used to actively transport protons across the inner mitochondrial membrane. The protons diffuse through ATP synthase down their concentration gradient and ATP is produced. The electrons and protons combine with oxygen and water is produced. Oxygen is the final electron acceptor.

> **Exam tip**
>
> Energy is *released* during respiration, not *produced*.

One of the ways of carrying out this practical involves using a dye such as methylene blue as an electron acceptor. The colour change can be seen easily and the time taken to change colour can be measured. The rate can be determined and used to investigate respiration because rate of colour change of the dye correlates to the rate of respiration.

As you will be investigating the effect of a factor on the rate of respiration, any factor that affects the enzymes involved in respiration or the proteins of the electron transfer chain will affect the overall rate of respiration. The factors that you could investigate are:

- temperature
- pH
- inhibitors

Another factor that would affect the rate of respiration is the respiratory substrate used.

> **Exam tip**
>
> Glucose and other sugars are not the only respiratory substrates that can be used to produce ATP — both lipids and proteins are potential sources of energy.

## Guidance through the practical

One of the first decisions that you need to make is which factor you are going to change and how you are going to change it. Having made this decision, you need to determine a suitable range for your independent variable. Temperature is an obvious choice as it is easy to vary using a water bath, and can be easily monitored and controlled. Make sure that you choose a range that will encompass the organism's optimum temperature.

Once you have chosen the factor that you are going to investigate, you must ensure that other factors that could affect the rate of respiration are controlled. You should also set up a control experiment to show that any change is due to respiration in the organisms. An example might be setting up an identical experiment, but using a boiled culture of organisms.

This practical requires you to use cultures of single-celled organisms, so a suspension of yeast is a popular choice. Alternatively, your teacher may provide you with a culture of non-pathogenic bacteria.

There are two main approaches to this investigation:

- Using a respirometer. Simple respirometers can be used to determine the rate of oxygen uptake in aerobic respiration, and production of carbon dioxide in both aerobic and anaerobic respiration.

- Using a dye or stain that changes colour when reduced. Methylene blue is a blue dye that can act as an artificial electron acceptor and will decolourise when reduced. The time taken to decolourise can be measured and used to calculate the rate. The higher the rate of respiration, the faster the dye will decolourise.

## Using a respirometer

As you can see from Figure 24, a simple respirometer has two key parts:

- An airtight tube or flask into which the living organisms can be placed together with a chemical, such as sodium hydroxide, that will absorb carbon dioxide.

- A capillary tube containing a drop of coloured liquid alongside a scale so that the distance travelled by the droplet can be measured.

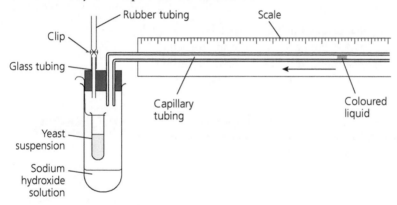

**Figure 24** A simple respirometer used to measure the rate of oxygen uptake by a yeast culture

When organisms respire aerobically, oxygen is taken up and carbon dioxide is released. If living organisms are in a sealed container and the carbon dioxide is absorbed, the uptake of oxygen will reduce the pressure inside the container as the oxygen taken from the air is not being replaced by carbon dioxide. A respirometer works on the principle that as the pressure inside the sealed container drops, it becomes lower than atmospheric pressure, causing a drop of coloured liquid to move along the capillary tube. The faster the rate of respiration, the further the bubble will move in a set period of time.

The tube containing the organisms could be immersed in water baths at different temperatures to investigate the effect of temperature.

## Using a dye as an electron acceptor

This method requires very little equipment and is a straightforward technique to carry out. The culture of single-celled organisms needs to be measured into a test tube along with glucose solution, then you need to measure the methylene blue into a second test tube. Both tubes should be left in the water bath at the required temperature for 5 minutes to equilibrate.

**Equilibrate** means 'to bring into equilibrium' and can be used in the context of a water bath to explain that a solution reaches the temperature of the water bath.

Variables that need to be controlled in this investigation are:

■ volume of culture of single-celled organisms
■ volume of glucose solution
■ volume of methylene blue

Once the tubes have reached the required temperature, you should add the methylene blue to the tube containing the organisms and glucose, shake the tube to mix the contents, then replace the tube in the water bath and start the stopwatch. Record the time taken for the dye to decolourise (for the blue colour to disappear).

Determining when the solution has completely decolourised is *subjective*. You should have a culture of organisms without methylene blue as a comparison so that you can see when the blue colour has disappeared.

You can repeat this for each temperature so that a mean can be calculated. You should then repeat for at least four other temperatures.

## Presentation of results from the practical

You will need to prepare a results table for your raw data before you start the practical. The factor that you are changing, such as temperature, will be in the first column, with units in the column heading only.

The subsequent columns in the table should be for your measurements of the distance moved by the drop of liquid. Depending on the apparatus, you may need columns for the start distance of the liquid, end distance of the liquid and the total distance moved. Alternatively, the respirometer that you use may allow you to reset the liquid to zero each time so that there would be no need to record the start and end positions of the bubble.

You will need a final column for processed data because this practical requires you to calculate *rate*. As rate is per unit time, you will need to record the distance travelled in a specific period of time, with the probable unit being $mm\,min^{-1}$. A better way of recording the rate would be to calculate the *volume* of oxygen taken up per minute ($mm^3\,min^{-1}$), as distance does not take the diameter of the capillary tube into account. See the maths skills box on page 48 for how to calculate this. An even better way of recording the data would be to calculate the rate of oxygen uptake per gram of organism ($mm^3\,min^{-1}\,g^{-1}$), in which case you would need to know the mass of yeast used in this practical (or other single-celled organism) used to make up the suspension.

If you have used the dye, you will still need to draw a table with the factor that you changed in the first column. The following columns will be for the time taken to decolourise in seconds (s), with enough columns for you to repeat each temperature and record the mean.

Process your mean time to give the rate for each temperature. This is calculated using 1/time, with a unit of $s^{-1}$.

Whichever method you follow, you can then plot a graph of your results. It will usually be a line graph because most of the factors you could investigate are continuous. (If you investigate different respiratory substrates, such as glucose, fructose and sucrose, you would draw a bar chart because the data are categoric.) The factor you investigate, for example temperature, will be on the *x*-axis and the rate on the *y*-axis. Draw a line of best fit, if appropriate, using the following rules:

**Practical tip**

Depending on your investigation, you could carry out a statistical test when analysing your results. A Student's *t*-test could be used to compare the means of two temperatures, or the correlation coefficient could be used to see if there is a relationship between temperature and rate.

- Ensure there are as many points on one side of the line as on the other.
- Draw a continuous line, using a sharp pencil.
- Do not **extrapolate** (extend the line beyond the first and last plotted points).
- Do not automatically ignore anomalous results.

## Analysis/evaluation of the results

Once you have plotted your graph, you should describe the pattern. You then need to explain your findings using your scientific knowledge. This is a good opportunity to make synoptic links — for example, you may need to discuss the enzymes and other proteins involved in respiration, and explain how they have been affected by the factor that you investigated.

### Focus on maths skills

#### Calculating surface areas and volumes

Calculating the surface area and volume of regular prisms, cylindrical prisms and spheres is one of the maths skills that may be assessed in the written exams. You need to learn the formulae shown in Figure 25 because they will not be provided in the exam.

For a regular prism:

$$\text{surface area} = 2wl + 2lh + 2hw$$

$$\text{volume} = lwh \ (l \times w \times h)$$

where $w$ = width, $l$ = length, and $h$ = height.

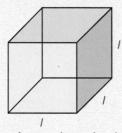

In the case of a regular cube, $l = w = h$ so:

$$\text{surface area} = 6l^2$$

$$\text{volume} = l^3$$

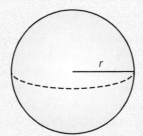

For a sphere:

$$\text{surface area} = 4\pi r^2$$

$$\text{volume} = \frac{4}{3}\pi r^3$$

where $r$ = radius and the value of $\pi$ is 3.14.

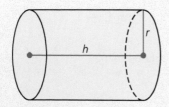

For a cylindrical prism:

$$\text{surface area} = 2\pi rh + 2\pi r^2$$

$$\text{volume} = \pi r^2 h$$

**Figure 25** Formulae for calculating surface areas and volumes

# Required practical 10

### The effect of an environmental variable on animal movement

## Background information

After studying the 'Stimuli and response' section of the specification, you will know that organisms respond to changes in their surroundings to increase their chances of survival. Motile organisms (organisms that can move) can show two types of simple response:

- **Taxes (plural of taxis)** — these are simple directional responses that involve an organism moving towards a favourable stimulus or away from an unfavourable stimulus. Movements towards a stimulus are positive taxes and movements away from a stimulus are negative taxes. There are different types of taxes depending on the stimulus. For example, chemotaxis is a response to a chemical stimulus and phototaxis is a response to light.

- **Kineses (plural of kinesis)** — these are non-directional responses that involve an organism changing its speed and turning frequency (Figure 26). When experiencing favourable conditions, an organism moves more slowly and turns more frequently so it remains in these favourable conditions. In unfavourable conditions, moving rapidly in a straight line increases an organism's chances of finding favourable conditions.

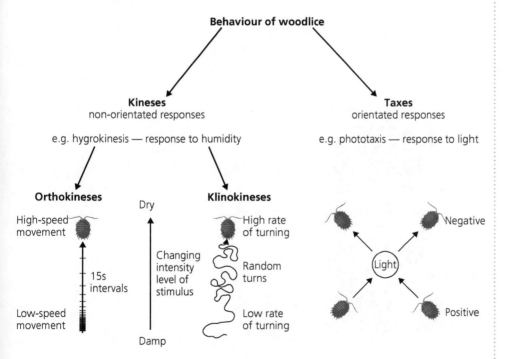

**Figure 26** Types of behaviour shown by woodlice including **orthokinesis** (when the speed of movement is dependent on the intensity of the stimulus) and **klinokinesis** (when the frequency or rate of turning is proportional to the stimulus)

A choice chamber is a shallow perspex container that generally has a base divided into four and a lid with small holes through which organisms can be placed. Figure 27 shows the typical structure of a choice chamber. Using a choice chamber allows you to create up to four different environmental conditions then, after a period of time, count the number of organisms in each section to determine their preferred environment.

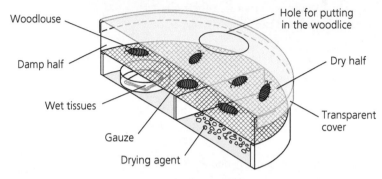

**Figure 27** Cross-section through a choice chamber, showing how dry and damp conditions could be created

Although no animal is specified in the title of the investigation, invertebrates such as woodlice and maggots are often used in schools and colleges because they are readily available and show a preference for certain conditions.

Woodlice are land crustaceans that are 10–15 mm in length and feed on rotten wood and vegetation. They have external gills for gas exchange (Figure 28), which are covered with a thin film of moisture, so prefer cool, damp conditions and can be found easily under stones and logs.

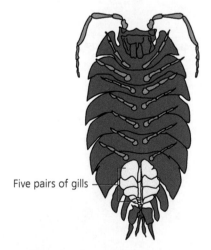

**Figure 28** Drawing of a woodlouse, showing the position of its gills

Maggots (Figure 29) are the larval stage of the European bluebottle and demonstrate negative phototaxis, behaviour that encourages them to burrow into their food (rotting food and faeces) and reduces their risk of predation and desiccation (drying out).

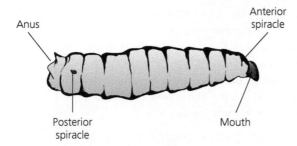

**Figure 29** Drawing of a maggot, showing the main body parts

## Guidance through the practical

Prior to completing this practical, a full risk assessment should be carried out either by you (as evidence for CPAC 3) or by your school or college. Handling animals can carry the risk of infection, and desiccants (drying agents) such as silica gel or anhydrous calcium chloride can be irritants. Referring to safety documents produced by CLEAPSS will inform you of appropriate control measures to take when handling these chemicals.

This is one of the few practicals that gives you the opportunity to handle living animals safely and ethically to measure their responses (ATh):

■ Handling living animals safely will minimise the risk of infection associated with them. You should avoid eating and drinking in the lab, cover open wounds with a plaster and wash your hands thoroughly with soap and warm water before leaving the lab.

■ Ethical handling of living animals refers to the way in which the animals are treated. Although they are simple organisms, they should still be treated with care and respect during the investigation.

If you have collected woodlice, then they should be returned to their habitat. Bluebottles are both a nuisance and carriers of disease, so the maggots should be killed humanely after use (by freezing for several days) and wrapped up securely before disposal.

When selecting the number of animals to use, bear in mind the number of conditions you are creating and the statistical test you intend to do. Statistical tests are discussed in more detail later in the practical. If you have four conditions, it makes sense to use a number of animals that is a multiple of four, to make subsequent calculations easier.

The practical title suggests the use of either a choice chamber or a maze. A choice chamber could be used to determine the preference of an organism for an environmental factor. You could investigate the preference for dry or humid conditions by adding a desiccant (dehydrating agent) such as silica gel or calcium chloride to one half of the chamber and damp filter paper or paper towel to the other half. You should leave the choice chamber to equilibrate for at least 5 minutes and check that the required conditions have been produced by testing with cobalt chloride strips, which are blue when dry and pink when moist. You should then insert the animals through the central hole, leave them for 5 minutes, then count and record the number of animals in each half. A preference for light or dark can also be investigated by covering one half with card, but you should ensure that the humidity and temperature are controlled.

**Practical tip**

The timings given for the investigation are for guidance only. You will need to adjust them depending on the animal you choose and its level of activity. Keep this time constant for any repeats.

You could also use a choice chamber to investigate kinesis by creating humid conditions in one half and dry conditions in the other. An animal could be inserted through a hole into the humid half and you could use a pen to trace its movement on the lid over a set period of time. Using this pen trace, you can measure the distance and count the number of turns made. If you repeat this process using a different animal each time and alternating humid and dry sections, you could then calculate the mean speed and the mean number of turns made in each condition.

You could make a simple maze out of paper or card, like the one shown in Figure 30, and use this to investigate taxes in animals. A food source could be placed at the end of either the left or right arm of the T-junction. You could then position an animal at position A and record whether it turns towards or away from the food source.

You should use a different animal each time and rub the inside of the maze with a cotton bud to remove any chemical trace left by the previous animal.

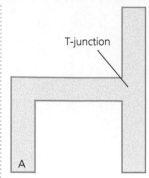

**Figure 30** A simple maze that could be used to investigate animal behaviour

## Presentation of results from the practical

A number of approaches have been described in the guidance above, but the presentation and analysis of results that follow will describe how to handle data from a choice chamber.

You should devise a suitable results table before starting the practical. This will probably be a simple table with the environmental condition in the first column and the number of animals present after 5 minutes in the second column.

A suitable number of repeats should be carried out and then the mean calculated and recorded in the final column.

## Analysis/evaluation of the results

### Chi-squared test

When analysing your results, you should use a statistical test to see if there is a significant difference in the distribution of the animals, or if any difference is just due to chance.

### Step 1 Write a null hypothesis

You should start with a null hypothesis, which could be: 'There is no significant difference between the number of woodlice found in dark and light areas.'

### Step 2 Choose a suitable statistical test and justify your choice

Use the flow chart given in Figure 31 (page 55) to help you choose a suitable test. You are collecting categoric data, so you would use the chi-squared ($\chi^2$) statistical test. For this practical, you are comparing your observed values with the expected values. The expected value is the number of organisms you would expect to find in each condition if they showed no preference for a particular environment. If you have two conditions, such as light and dark, you would expect to find an equal number in each section.

A **null hypothesis** is a testable statement that there is no significant difference between the samples being tested.

## Step 3 Calculate the test statistic

You then need to calculate chi-squared using the formula:

$$\chi^2 = \sum \frac{(O-E)^2}{E}$$

where $O$ = your **observed** values (the number of animals that you counted in each section) and $E$ = your **expected** values (an equal number of animals in each section). The easiest way to work through this calculation is by using a table, as shown in Table 7.

**Table 7** How to calculate chi-squared — a worked example

| Environmental condition | Observed number of animals ($O$) | Expected number of animals ($E$) | $(O-E)$ | $(O-E)^2$ | $\dfrac{(O-E)^2}{E}$ |
|---|---|---|---|---|---|
| Dark | 11 | 7 | 4 | 16 | 2.29 |
| Light | 3 | 7 | −4 | 16 | 2.29 |
| | | | | | $\Sigma = 4.58$ |

## Step 4 Interpret the test statistic

Once you have calculated chi-squared, you need to look up the critical value of chi-squared in a table of probability. The number of degrees of freedom is your number of categories minus 1. The example above only has two categories, light and dark, so the number of degrees of freedom is 1. The critical value of chi-squared for 1 degree of freedom is 3.84 at the $p = 0.05$ level.

In the example above, the calculated value of chi-squared is 4.58, which is greater than the critical value of 3.84 at 1 degree of freedom.

If your value of chi-squared is *greater* than the critical value, then you *reject* the null hypothesis. There is *less* than 5% probability that the difference in distribution is due to chance. This means that there *is* a significant difference in the distribution of the animals, and you may be expected to suggest reasons for this difference.

If your value of chi-squared is *lower* than the critical value, then you *accept* the null hypothesis. There is *more* than a 5% probability that the difference in distribution is due to chance. This means that there is no significant difference in the distribution of the animals.

### Focus on maths skills

#### Statistical tests

One of the maths skills that you may be assessed on is your ability to select and use a statistical test. There are three statistical tests in the specification: the chi-squared test, the Student's $t$-test and 'a test of correlation' (e.g. Spearman's rank correlation test).

The chi-squared test should be used if you are comparing frequencies of categoric data. This test is used to analyse the results of genetic crosses, because you can compare observed ratios with the ratios predicted from genetic diagrams. It is also useful for analysing data on animal behaviour, for example, whether a species of butterfly has a preference for a certain flower colour.

**Exam tip**

Lay out any calculations clearly and annotate fully. This may gain marks for your method, even if your final answer is incorrect.

**Practical tip**

$\Sigma$ means 'the sum of', so you need to add the values in the final column.

**Exam tip**

There are different significance levels, but the $p = 0.05$ level is the one you will use. If the probability of the results being due to chance is less than or equal to $p = 0.05$ (5% or 1 in 20), then the difference is significant.

The Student's *t*-test is used when comparing the means of two sets of data. An example of when you might use this test is when comparing the mean diameter of limpets on the upper and lower sections of a rocky shore.

To calculate the value of *t*, you need to know:
- the means of each sample ($\bar{x}_1$ and $\bar{x}_2$)
- the number of measurements in each sample ($n_1$ and $n_2$)
- the variances of each sample (the variance is the square of the standard deviation)

A correlation coefficient is used when you are looking for associations between two sets of data. This is a useful statistical test when you are carrying out fieldwork investigations where, for example, you may be looking for a correlation between the distribution of a species and an abiotic factor. The correlation coefficient recommended by AQA is Spearman's rank, but others may be used.

Although you are expected to have used these statistical tests and to have a sound understanding of them, *you will not be asked to perform calculations using them in the exam papers*.

In the AS exams, you may be asked to *formulate* a null hypothesis for a practical that you have carried out or for a given experiment, and in the A-level exams you may be asked to *evaluate* a null hypothesis.

Your ability to *select* an appropriate statistical test and then *justify* this selection may be assessed in the AS exams, whereas the A-level exams may also ask you to *evaluate* another investigator's choice of statistical test. Figure 31 shows a flow chart that may help you choose an appropriate statistical test.

At AS you may be given a probability value and be expected to *interpret* whether the results are due to chance. At A-level you may be expected to *interpret* a probability value, with a statement about whether to accept or reject the null hypothesis using $p = 0.05$, as well as *evaluating* conclusions about data. At A-level you may also be given an extract from a table of probability (similar to the one shown in Table 8) and be expected to find a probability value for the appropriate number of degrees of freedom. For example, the critical value for *t* at the 5% ($p = 0.05$) level and with 2 degrees of freedom is 4.30.

**Table 8** An extract from a statistical test table for values of *t*

| Degrees of freedom | Significance level | | | |
|---|---|---|---|---|
| | 10% ($p = 0.10$) | 5% ($p = 0.05$) | 1% ($p = 0.01$) | 0.1% ($p = 0.001$) |
| 1 | 6.31 | 12.71 | 63.66 | 636.62 |
| 2 | 2.92 | 4.30 | 9.93 | 31.60 |
| 3 | 2.35 | 3.18 | 5.84 | 12.94 |

➜

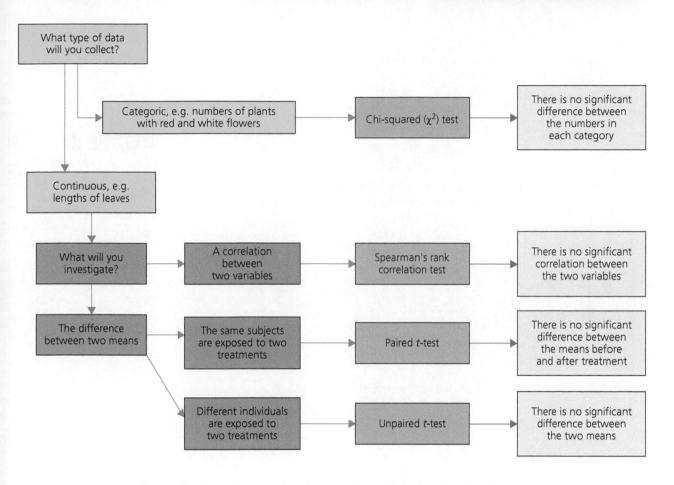

**Figure 31** A flow chart to use when deciding which statistical test to use

### Student's t-test

A student investigates the hypothesis that there is a difference between the diameter of limpets on the upper section of a rocky shore in Aberystwyth and those on the lower section of the shore. He measures the diameter of 12 limpets on the upper shore and 12 limpets on the lower shore and then works out the mean limpet diameter for each section of the shore. He then wants to carry out a statistical test to see if there is a significant difference between the mean diameters.

#### Step 1 Write a null hypothesis

A null hypothesis for this investigation could be: 'There is no significant difference between the mean diameters of limpets from the upper and lower shore.'

#### Step 2 Select a suitable statistical test and justify your choice

Referring to the flow chart in Figure 31, diameter is a continuous variable and the difference between two means is being compared. In this investigation, different groups of individuals are exposed to two treatments (the upper shore and the lower shore), so the student uses the unpaired t-test.

# Skills Guidance

## Step 3 Calculate the test statistic

The value of $t$ is calculated using the formula:

$$t = \frac{\overline{x}_1 - \overline{x}_2}{\sqrt{\dfrac{s_1^2}{n_1} + \dfrac{s_2^2}{n_2}}}$$

where:
- $\overline{x}_1$ and $\overline{x}_2$ are the means for the upper and lower shore
- $s_1^2$ and $s_2^2$ are the variances for the upper and lower shore
- $n_1$ and $n_2$ are the number of limpets measured on the upper and lower shores

The results from the investigation are shown in Table 9.

**Table 9** Data on limpet diameter from the upper and lower shores

|  | Upper shore | Lower shore |
|---|---|---|
| Number of limpets measured ($n$) | 12 | 12 |
| Mean diameter/mm | 13.2 | 7.9 |
| Standard deviation ($s$)/mm | 2.17 | 1.16 |
| Variance ($s^2$) | 4.71 (to 2 d.p.) | 1.35 (to 2 d.p.) |

The figures from Table 9 can be substituted into the formula to give a value for $t$:

$$t = \frac{13.2 - 7.9}{\sqrt{\left(\dfrac{4.71}{12} + \dfrac{1.35}{12}\right)}}$$

$$t = \frac{5.3}{\sqrt{0.505}}$$

$$t = \frac{5.3}{0.7106}$$

$$t = 7.458 \text{ (to 3 d.p.)}$$

## Step 4 Interpret the test statistic

Once the value of $t$ has been calculated, the critical value of $t$ is found for $(n_1 + n_2) - 2$ degrees of freedom. As 12 measurements were taken at each site, the number of degrees of freedom for the worked example is 22. Table 10 shows an extract from a statistical table for values of $t$.

**Table 10** Critical values of $t$

| Number of degrees of freedom | Significance level | | | |
|---|---|---|---|---|
|  | $p = 0.10$ (10%) | $p = 0.05$ (5%) | $p = 0.01$ (1%) | $p = 0.001$ (0.1%) |
| 22 | 1.717 | 2.074 | 2.819 | 3.792 |

**Practical tip**

Although standard deviation can be calculated manually, it is expected that you will use a calculator. If you are not sure how to do this, find someone with the same type of calculator as you and ask them to show you how to do it, or check in your instruction manual.

The calculated value of *t* of 7.458 is much greater than the critical value of 3.792 at $p = 0.001$ (0.1%). This means that the probability of the difference between the means occurring by chance is less than 0.1%, so it is therefore *highly unlikely* that the difference between the two means could have occurred by chance. The *null hypothesis is rejected* and the difference between the mean diameters of the limpets is significant.

# Required practical 11

## Using a calibration curve to identify an unknown concentration

## Background information

This practical is linked to the specification section 'Control of blood glucose concentration', which requires you to know the roles of the liver and hormones, including insulin, glucagon and adrenaline.

**Glycogenesis** is the conversion of glucose to glycogen. **Gluconeogenesis** is the production of glucose from non-carbohydrate sources such as amino acids. **Glycogenolysis** is the breakdown of glycogen to glucose.

### Exam tip

There are many similar-sounding words in this section that students sometimes get mixed up. Glucagon is a hormone and glycogen is a storage polysaccharide. You also need to learn the difference between glycogenesis, gluconeogenesis and glycogenolysis.

You should also know the causes and control of type I and type II diabetes. There are a number of **signs** and **symptoms** of diabetes, with glucose in the urine being one of the signs.

Normally, the urine contains no glucose because it is all reabsorbed in the proximal convoluted tubule, but high levels of glucose in the blood can lead to glycosuria (glucose in the urine). Glycosuria leads to increased water loss in the urine, so frequent urination is a symptom of diabetes. The presence of glucose in urine can be shown using reagent test strips, such as Diastix®, which are dipped into urine and change colour to indicate the concentration of glucose present. In this practical you will use Benedict's reagent to test a solution made up by the technician to resemble urine. This required practical does *not* require you to test real urine!

**Signs** of a disease can be seen or measured, whereas **symptoms** are felt by the patient. A high temperature and rash are signs, whereas pain and tiredness are symptoms.

The Benedict's test is a test for reducing sugars, which includes all monosaccharides and some disaccharides. Sucrose is a disaccharide and is not a reducing sugar. Benedict's solution contains copper(II) sulfate, which is reduced to copper(I) oxide when heated with a reducing sugar. This forms an insoluble red precipitate and so the presence of a reducing sugar can be seen by a colour change.

The Benedict's test can be used **quantitatively** because the mass of precipitate formed correlates to the concentration of reducing sugar present. The test can also be used **semi-quantitatively** because the colour obtained gives an indication of the concentration of reducing sugar present. The solution remains blue in the absence of reducing sugar, then changes colour to green, yellow, orange or brick-red with increasing reducing sugar concentration, as illustrated in Figure 32.

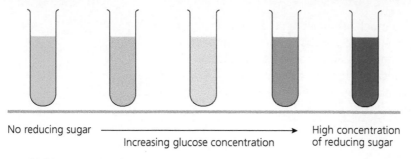

No reducing sugar ———————————————————→ High concentration
of reducing sugar

Increasing glucose concentration

**Figure 32** Diagram showing the approximate colours of Benedict's reagent with a range of different glucose concentrations

## Guidance through the practical

This is a straightforward practical and two of the key skills — using glassware for dilutions (ATc) and using a colorimeter to record quantitative measurements (ATb) — have already been covered in detail in required practicals 3 and 4. Additionally, you will use Benedict's solution to identify the presence of a reducing sugar (ATf).

The first stage of this practical is preparing your dilution series using a stock glucose solution and distilled water. The stock solution and the distilled water will be two of your test samples, and you should prepare at least four intermediate concentrations. If you were given a stock solution of $10.0\,\text{mmol}\,\text{dm}^{-3}$ concentration, you could use this to prepare intermediate concentrations of 2.0, 4.0, 6.0 and $8.0\,\text{mmol}\,\text{dm}^{-3}$.

Once you have made your dilutions, you need to carry out the Benedict's test on each sample. This involves adding Benedict's solution to your test samples and heating them in a water bath of hot water (about 70°C). There are a number of variables that you need to control to allow comparison of the final colours:

- volume of each test sample
- volume of Benedict's solution
- temperature of water bath
- time in the water bath

You should now have at least six tubes of known glucose concentration that have been heated with Benedict's solution and then left to cool. You should also have at least one unknown sample of fake urine (prepared by your teacher or technician) that has also been heated with Benedict's solution.

The second stage of the practical is taking the absorbance readings, using a colorimeter.

You can remove the precipitate by filtering each solution into a clean test tube labelled with the glucose concentration. Depending on the colorimeter that you are using, you may be able to leave the solutions in the test tubes, or you may need to transfer the contents of each tube to a clean cuvette.

When setting up the colorimeter, you will need to use the contents of the tube with $0.0\,\text{mmol}\,\text{dm}^{-3}$ glucose tested with Benedict's solution as your blank, not just distilled water. Record the absorbance of each solution in your results table.

## Presentation of results from the practical

Draw a results table with the concentration of glucose solution/mmol dm$^{-3}$ in the first column and absorbance in the second column. Remember that there are no units for absorbance because it is a ratio.

You then need to plot a graph of your results, with concentration of glucose solution on the *x*-axis and absorbance on the *y*-axis. Draw a suitable line of best fit through your points. You may find that it is a straight line, or it may be a curve, depending on the concentrations of glucose used. The graph is still called a **calibration curve** even if it is a straight line.

In this practical, if you *have not filtered* the solutions, you would expect absorbance to *increase* (or percentage light transmission to *decrease*) as the concentration of glucose *increases*. This is because at a high glucose concentration a greater mass of precipitate would form due to the reaction between the glucose and the copper sulfate ions, and more light would be absorbed by the solution.

If you *have filtered* the solutions to remove the precipitate, then absorbance would *decrease* as the concentration of glucose *increases*. At low concentrations of glucose, few Cu(II) ions are reduced to Cu(I) so the solution remains a darker blue and gives a higher absorbance. More reduction of Cu(II) at higher glucose concentrations produces a lighter blue solution and so a lower absorbance.

## Analysis/evaluation of the results

Once you have plotted your calibration curve, you can use it to find the glucose concentration of your unknown solution. Find the absorbance of the unknown solution on the *y*-axis and read across until you reach the curve; then read down to find the value of the intercept on the *x*-axis.

Figure 33 shows that an unknown solution has an absorbance of 1.00. Reading across to the curve and then down to the *x*-intercept, the glucose concentration of the unknown solution is found to be 3.7%.

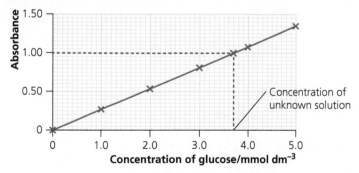

**Figure 33** How to use a calibration curve to determine the *x*-axis intercept

**Practical tip**

When you are using a calibration curve to determine an unknown value, use a ruler to draw dashed lines from the measured value on the *y*-axis to the curve, then from the curve down to the intercept on the *x*-axis.

## Focus on maths skills

### Representing uncertainty

When plotting a point on a graph, there is always a level of uncertainty. You may be plotting a mean value, in which case your level of uncertainty depends on the values used to calculate the mean, and the presence or absence of anomalous results.

**Range bars** are the simplest way of showing the spread of data around the mean. The maximum and minimum values used to calculate the mean are marked above and below the plotted point using small lines, and the two lines are joined by a vertical line through the plotted point.

**Error bars** are drawn in exactly the same way as range bars, but may be shown as plus and minus one standard deviation above and below the plotted point (or bar), as shown in Figure 34. Using the standard deviation rather than the range is preferable because calculating standard deviation still shows the spread of data around the mean, but minimises the effect of extreme values. The longer the error bars, the greater the spread of data around the mean.

If you draw a line of best fit that does not go through each plotted point, then it should be drawn within the error bars.

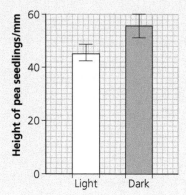

**Figure 34** A graph showing the height of pea seedlings grown in the light and in the dark. Error bars have been included to show the spread of data around the mean

# Required practical 12

### The effect of environmental factors on species distribution

## Background information

The location chosen for this practical activity will depend on the amount of time available and the proximity of your school or college to a suitable site. Some schools and colleges visit specialist fieldwork centres, with popular choices for this type of investigation being sand dunes and rocky shores.

The study of the interactions between organisms and their environment is called **ecology**. The environment includes both abiotic (non-living) and biotic (living) factors. Abiotic factors include:

- light intensity
- temperature
- oxygen concentration
- pH

Biotic factors include:

- predation
- competition
- disease

You will have studied the effects of these abiotic and biotic factors on populations in the 'Populations in ecosystems' section of the specification.

Your choice of sampling technique will depend on the factor you are investigating and the hypothesis you have developed, but the two main techniques are random sampling and systematic sampling.

## Random sampling

This is a technique designed to remove **sampling bias**. The person carrying out the investigation may deliberately or unconsciously make a biased choice, for example putting a quadrat down on a patch of grass with the most daisies. One random sampling technique is to divide the area being investigated into a grid using two tape measures as axes. Random numbers can be generated using a table of random numbers, or a random number generator on a calculator. These random numbers can be used as coordinates, with a sample being taken where the coordinates intersect, as shown in Figure 35. Random sampling does not involve throwing a quadrat over your shoulder without looking!

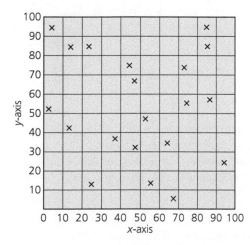

**Figure 35** How to place quadrats using random number coordinates

**Exam tip**

Learn the key definitions for this topic. Students are often unclear on the meanings of:

- population
- community
- ecosystem
- habitat
- niche

**Exam tip**

When referring to random numbers in an exam, state *how* you will generate the random numbers.

### Systematic sampling

This technique involves taking samples at regular intervals and is useful if you are investigating a correlation, or if you are looking at the stages of succession. An example of a systematic sampling technique is an interrupted belt transect (Figure 36). A tape measure could be laid across the ground and then samples taken at regular intervals, for example every 1 m or every 10 m (depending on the total distance to be covered).

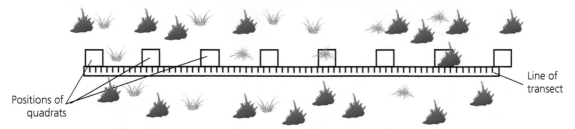

Positions of quadrats

Line of transect

**Figure 36** How to carry out an interrupted belt transect

Both techniques described above may require the use of a quadrat (Figure 37). This is a square frame made of metal or plastic, usually $0.25\,\text{m}^2$, that is divided into smaller squares and can be used to sample plants or non-motile organisms. The number of organisms could be counted, or the percentage cover could be estimated.

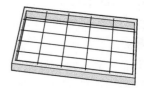

**Figure 37** A typical wooden-framed quadrat

## Guidance through the practical

This is an open-ended investigation, which lends itself to a full planning activity that could provide evidence for all of the CPAC. Unlike some of the required practicals, very little equipment is necessary and the investigation could be carried out completely independently in your garden or a nearby park.

During this practical, the main skill you will develop is the use of sampling techniques in fieldwork (AT k). The sampling technique you choose will depend on your hypothesis, and on your choice of both environmental factor and organism. You need to decide if random sampling or systematic sampling is more appropriate for your investigation.

Once you have decided on a sampling technique, you need to choose a sample size. You need a suitable number of samples for statistical analysis. A large sample size will also minimise the effect of anomalies and give more representative measurements.

The size of the species being investigated and the size of the area being investigated will affect the *size of quadrat* that you choose. The area being sampled and the available time will determine the *number of quadrats* that you include in your sample, but you could carry out some preliminary work to determine the optimum quadrat number to use.

As you are investigating the effect of an environmental factor, you also need a method of measuring this factor. For example, a light meter could be used to measure light intensity, the pH of soil or water could be measured using a pH probe, and nitrate test strips could be used to determine the concentration of soil nitrates.

Some possible investigation titles include:
- The effect of wind speed on the distribution of marram grass on a sand dune
- The effect of light intensity on the distribution of daisies on a lawn
- The effect of oxygen concentration on invertebrate distribution in a river

## Presentation of results from the practical

Preparing a results table prior to this investigation is important, because you will be outside collecting the data. It may be a good idea to prepare a table for your raw data on a piece of paper attached to a clipboard rather than risking getting your lab book wet or dirty. Weatherproof paper or a plastic wallet will allow you to keep a clear record of your data in adverse weather conditions.

Different types of graph may be drawn; you should select the one most appropriate for your investigation.

You may choose to draw a bar chart if the independent variable is categoric. As the independent variable is not continuous, the bars should not touch.

## Analysis/evaluation of the results

You will need to carry out a statistical analysis of your results to find out if your results are significant. If you find that your results are significant, then you should research the reasons for them and explain your observations using your biological knowledge. If your results are not statistically significant, you should explore possible reasons for this, with an evaluation of your methodology and possible improvements to your investigation.

This analysis provides an excellent opportunity for you to make synoptic links:
- If you have investigated temperature, you could discuss the effect on enzymes.
- For light intensity, you could make links to photosynthesis.
- Salt concentration could be linked to osmosis and xerophytic adaptations.
- Nitrate concentration could be discussed with reference to the nitrogen cycle, protein synthesis and growth.

### Focus on maths skills

#### Correlation

Scatter diagrams or scattergrams are used to identify a correlation between two variables (Figure 38) and you may be assessed on your ability to interpret them. The relationship between the two variables could be:
- no correlation — there is no relationship between the two variables
- positive correlation — as one variable increases, the other variable increases
- negative correlation — as one variable increases, the other variable decreases

→

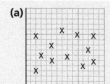 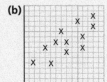 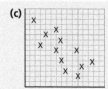

**Figure 38** Scattergrams showing three possible trends: (a) no correlation; (b) positive correlation; (c) negative correlation

Just because there is a **correlation** between two variables, it does not mean that there is a **causal** link. There may be a correlation between ice cream sales and cases of hay fever, but that does not mean that ice cream causes hay fever.

### The correlation coefficient

When you plan an investigation looking for a correlation or association between two variables, you start with a **hypothesis**, a testable statement. For example:
- There is a correlation between the distance from the strand line on a rocky shore and the number of bladders present on bladder wrack (a type of seaweed).
- There is a correlation between the distance from the strand line and the concentration of nitrate in the soil on the sand dunes.
- There is a correlation between the percentage cover of marram grass on the sand dunes and the wind speed.
- There is a relationship between the distance from the upper section of a rocky shore and the diameter of limpets.

Once you have completed your investigation and collected your data, you need to carry out a statistical test to determine whether or not the correlation is significant.

A student hypothesises that there is a correlation between wind speed and the percentage cover of marram grass on the sand dunes in Aberystwyth. At 12 randomly selected points in the dunes, she uses a quadrat to estimate the percentage cover of marram grass and an anemometer to measure the wind speed. The following steps describe how to analyse the data that she collects.

### Step 1 Write a null hypothesis

The **null hypothesis** states that there is no relationship or correlation. For example: 'There is no correlation between the percentage cover of marram grass on the sand dunes and wind speed.'

### Step 2 Select a statistical test and justify your choice

Choose a suitable statistical test using the flow chart in Figure 31 (page 55). As you are looking for a correlation between two variables, you will use the **Spearman's rank** correlation test. This test shows the strength and direction (positive or negative) of a relationship between two variables.

### Step 3 Calculate the test statistic

As you are using Spearman's rank correlation test, you need to calculate the correlation coefficient using the formula:

$$r_s = 1 - \frac{6\sum D^2}{n^3 - n}$$

**Exam tip**

Do not write casual instead of **causal**.

**Practical tip**

Spearman's rank is one type of correlation test, but other statistical tests can be used, for example Pearson's product moment correlation test. In each case you calculate a correlation coefficient.

where:

■ $r_s$ = correlation coefficient
■ $\Sigma$ = sum of
■ $D$ = difference between the ranks
■ $n$ = number of pairs of measurements

Table 11 shows a straightforward method of presenting your results when you are calculating the Spearman's rank correlation coefficient.

**Table 11** How to calculate the Spearman's rank correlation coefficient — a worked example

| Wind speed/m s$^{-1}$ | Rank wind speed | Percentage cover of marram grass | Rank percentage cover | Difference between ranks ($D$) | $D^2$ |
|---|---|---|---|---|---|
| 1.4 | 4 | 80 | 4 | 0 (4 – 4) | 0 |
| 1.2 | 6 | 100 | 1 | 5 (6 – 1) | 25 |
| 0.2 | 12 | 60 | 7.5 | 4.5 (12 – 7.5) | 20.25 |
| 1.3 | 5 | 70 | 6 | –1 | 1 |
| 0.3 | 10.5 | 40 | 9 | 1.5 | 2.25 |
| 0.3 | 10.5 | 20 | 11 | –0.5 | 0.25 |
| 1.9 | 2 | 80 | 4 | –2 | 4 |
| 0.6 | 8 | 30 | 10 | –2 | 4 |
| 2.8 | 1 | 80 | 4 | –3 | 9 |
| 1.8 | 3 | 90 | 2 | 1 | 1 |
| 0.7 | 7 | 60 | 7.5 | –0.5 | 0.25 |
| 0.4 | 9 | 0 | 12 | –3 | 9 |
| | | | | | $\Sigma D^2$ = 76 |

1 Rank the wind speed by giving the highest value a '1', the second highest a '2' and so on. If you have two values the same, like 0.3 m s$^{-1}$ in Table 11, they 'share' ranks 10 and 11 and are both given a rank of 10.5. The next value in Table 11, 0.2 m s$^{-1}$, then takes rank 12.
2 Rank the percentage cover of marram grass, again giving the highest percentage cover a rank of '1'. If you have three values the same, like 80% in Table 11, they share ranks 3, 4 and 5 and are all given ranks of 4 (the mean of 3, 4 and 5). The next value, 70%, takes rank 6.
3 Find the difference between the ranks ($D$) by subtracting each rank for percentage marram grass cover from the rank for wind speed.
4 Calculate $D^2$.
5 Add up all of the values of $D^2$ ($\Sigma D^2$) = 76
6 Multiply $\Sigma D^2$ by 6 ($6\Sigma D^2$) = 6 × 76 = 456
7 Calculate $n^3 - n$ = $12^3$ – 12 = 1728 – 12 = 1716
8 Find $6\Sigma D^2/(n^3 - n)$ = 456/1716 = 0.2657342
9 Find $1 - [6\Sigma D^2/(n^3 - n)]$ = 0.7342657 = 0.734 (to 3 d.p.)

Don't forget the last step. This is commonly overlooked by students.

**Practical tip**

When you are ranking values, write a list of numbers and cross out each number as you use it in your ranking so that you do not accidentally use the same rank too many times. This is particularly useful if you have values that are the same.

➔

# Skills Guidance

You have now calculated the test statistic and have a value of 0.734 for the correlation coefficient. Your answer should be given to three decimal places because critical values in probability tables are usually given to three decimal places.

## Step 4 Interpreting the test statistic

Your calculated value of $r_s$ will be between −1 (a perfect negative correlation) and +1 (a perfect positive correlation). The closer your calculated value is to 0, the weaker the correlation.

Once you have calculated the test statistic, you need to look up the critical value of Spearman's rank for the number of pairs of measurements ($n$). Table 12 shows an extract from a probability table.

**Table 12** Critical values for Spearman's rank correlation coefficient

| Number of pairs of measurements ($n$) | Significance level | | | |
|---|---|---|---|---|
| | $p = 0.10$ (10%) | $p = 0.05$ (5%) | $p = 0.01$ (1%) | $p = 0.001$ (0.1%) |
| 10 | 0.564 | 0.648 | 0.794 | 0.903 |
| 12 | 0.503 | 0.587 | 0.727 | 0.846 |
| 14 | 0.464 | 0.538 | 0.679 | 0.802 |

There were 12 pairs of measurements in the worked example, so the critical value for $r_s$ for 12 pairs of measurements at the 5% level ($p = 0.05$) is 0.587.

The calculated value of 0.734 is *greater than* the critical value of 0.587 at the 5% level, so the *null hypothesis is rejected*. There *is a correlation* between wind speed and the percentage cover of marram grass.

The value of 0.734 falls between the critical values for $p = 0.01$ and $p = 0.001$ for 12 pairs of measurements, so there is a probability of between $p = 0.01$ (1%) and $p = 0.001$ (0.1%) that this result occurred by chance.

As the calculated value is a positive number, it indicates a positive correlation, so as wind speed increases the percentage cover of marram grass also increases.

If you have established that there is a correlation, you can investigate whether or not there is a **causal relationship**. Just because two variables are linked, this does not prove that one causes the other. There could be a third variable that has not been investigated.

# Questions & Answers

## The exams

At AS there are two 1½-hour examination papers, each worth 50% of the total AS grade. Papers 1 and 2 assess any of the content from topics 1–4, including practical skills. At A-level there are three 2-hour exam papers. Paper 1 assesses any of the content from topics 1–4, paper 2 assesses the content from topics 5–8 and paper 3 assesses any content from the specification. Papers 1 and 2 are worth 35% each and paper 3 is worth 30%. Paper 3 includes questions requiring you to critically analyse experimental data. It also includes a 25-mark essay from a choice of two titles.

## About this section

This section contains questions on some of the required practicals. These may appear in any of the papers in both the AS and the A-level exams. They are written in the same style as the questions in the exam so they will give you an indication of what you can expect. After each question there are answers by two different students.

Comments on the questions are preceded by the icon ⓔ. They offer tips on what you need to do to gain full marks. All student responses are followed by examiner's comments, indicated by the icon ⓔ, which highlight where credit is due. In the weaker answers, they also point out areas for improvement, specific problems and common errors such as lack of clarity, irrelevance, misinterpretation of the question and mistaken meanings of terms.

## Question 1 The effect of pH on starch hydrolysis

A student investigated the effect of pH on the time taken by amylase to hydrolyse starch. The student:

1 added amylase and starch suspension to a test tube containing a buffer solution at pH 3

2 stood the test tube in a water bath and started a stopwatch

3 took samples at regular intervals and tested them with iodine solution

4 continued to take samples until a blue-black colour no longer appeared, and then recorded the time

5 repeated steps 1–4 using buffers at pH 5, 7, 9 and 11

**(a)** The student controlled the temperature. State *two* other variables that she should have controlled. (2 marks)

ⓔ This question just requires you to state two variables, but these should be *other than* temperature, which is given in the question.

**(b)** Describe how the student could have monitored the temperature. (2 marks)

ⓔ Note that there are 2 marks for this question. Which piece of equipment would you use *and* how would you use it?

**(c)** The student maintained the temperature at 30°C. Explain why the rate of starch hydrolysis would be faster at 40°C. (2 marks)

ⓔ The command word is *explain*, so this question requires you to use your knowledge of collision theory from topic 1: Biological molecules.

**(d)** The student took samples until the blue-black colour no longer appeared. How could she have ensured that her decision was consistent? (1 mark)

ⓔ You need to describe what you could compare each sample against when determining the end-point.

The student calculated the rate of reaction and plotted a graph of the results, as shown in Figure 1.

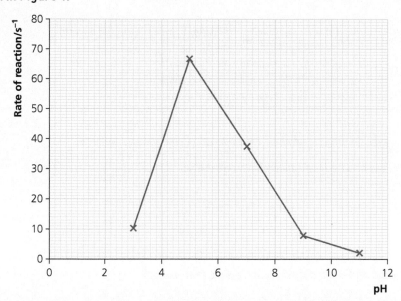

**Figure 1** Graph to show the effect of pH on the rate of starch hydrolysis by amylase

**(e)** Explain why she joined the points with straight lines rather than drawing a line of best fit. (1 mark)

ⓔ Look at the intervals between each pH that the student tested.

**(f)** The student concluded that pH 5 was the optimum pH for this enzyme because the results show that the rate was highest at pH 5. Explain why this conclusion may not be valid. (2 marks)

**ⓔ** The student has only found pH 5 to have the fastest rate of the pHs that she tested. Think about a further investigation that would give an optimum pH closer to the true value.

> **Student A**
> **(a)** concentration of amylase and temperature

**ⓔ** **1/2 marks awarded** Temperature does need to be controlled, but this variable is given in the question.

> **(b)** She could stand a thermometer in the water bath and check the temperature every 10 minutes to make sure it stays constant.

**ⓔ** **2/2 marks awarded** Student A clearly describes a method that could be used to monitor the temperature. The answer does not need to specify 10-minute intervals as long as the temperature is checked regularly.

> **(c)** The starch and amylase have more kinetic energy at higher temperatures so there are more successful collisions and more enzyme–substrate complexes form.

**ⓔ** **2/2 marks awarded** This answer clearly explains the effect of a higher temperature on the enzyme and substrate, and why this would increase rate.

> **(d)** She could have compared the colour of each sample to a sample of reaction mixture that has gone to completion and been tested with iodine solution.

**ⓔ** **1/1 mark awarded** This is an excellent answer that would allow the determination of a consistent end-point.

> **(e)** She cannot be sure of the intermediate values, so she should join each point with a straight, ruled line.

**ⓔ** **1/1 mark awarded** This is an excellent answer.

> **(f)** The student needs to repeat the investigation using pH 4, 6, 8 and 10.

**ⓔ** **1/2 marks awarded** Student A has realised that intermediate values need to be tested, but the optimum cannot be above 7 as the rate is decreasing. A better answer would suggest testing around pH 5, for example pH 4, 4.5, 5.5 and 6.

(a) volume of amylase and pH

*e* 1/2 marks awarded Although pH is a factor that affects the rate of an enzyme-controlled reaction, in this investigation pH is the independent variable.

(b) She could check the temperature using a thermometer.

*e* 1/2 marks awarded There needs to be the idea of taking the temperature at regular intervals to gain the second marking point.

(c) The enzyme and substrate molecules move around faster and so the rate is faster.

*e* 0/2 marks awarded This answer lacks scientific terminology — there is no reference to 'kinetic energy', 'collisions' or 'enzyme–substrate complexes'. It also repeats the stem of the question rather than explaining *why* the rate is faster.

(d) The student could mix amylase with water and test with iodine solution, and then compare her samples with this colour.

*e* 1/1 mark awarded This is a good suggestion that would also allow a consistent end-point to be determined.

(e) The student should draw a curve.

*e* 0/1 mark awarded Student B is confused because many graphs show the effect of pH on the rate of an enzyme-controlled reaction as a curve. This does not answer the question.

(f) The student needs to repeat the investigation using a bigger range of pH.

*e* 0/2 marks awarded A bigger range suggests using pH below 3 and above 11, which would not provide a more accurate value for the optimum pH.

# Question 2 Preparing an onion root tip squash

A student removed the tip from an onion root and put it into $5\,mol\,dm^{-3}$ solution of hydrochloric acid to kill the cells. He then followed instructions to separate and stain the cells. He placed a coverslip on top of the root tip and pressed down firmly, then viewed the slide using an optical microscope.

Figure 2 shows some of the cells he viewed.

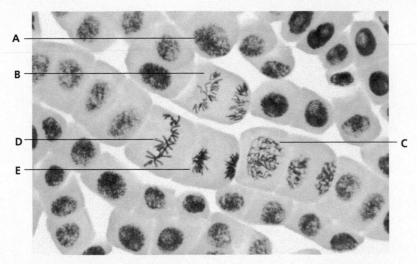

**Figure 2** Cells from the tip of a plant root as seen using an optical microscope

**(a)** Cell A is undergoing interphase. State what happens to the DNA during interphase. (1 mark)

ⓔ Remember that interphase is a stage of the cell cycle and *not* a stage of mitosis.

**(b)** Name the stages of mitosis shown by cells B, C, D and E. (4 marks)

ⓔ As well as knowing what happens at each stage of mitosis, you need to familiarise yourself with diagrams and photos of each stage.

**(c)** Explain why the student added a drop of stain to the slide. (1 mark)

ⓔ There are many different stains used in the preparation of slides, but they all have the same general function.

**(d)** Explain why the coverslip was pressed down firmly. (1 mark)

ⓔ A root tip would be a piece of tissue consisting of many layers of cells. What would you need to do if you wanted to view individual cells?

**(e)** Suggest why the student handled the hydrochloric acid with caution. (1 mark)

ⓔ Look at the concentration of the hydrochloric acid. How does this compare with the concentrations you may have used during your other practical activities? The unit $mol\,dm^{-3}$ (moles per $dm^3$) is also written as 'M'.

---

**Student A**

**(a)** The DNA is replicated.

ⓔ **1/1 mark awarded** Correct — the mass of DNA doubles during interphase, which takes up most of the cell cycle, and is followed by nuclear division and cytokinesis.

**(b)** B — anaphase, C — prophase, D — metaphase, E — telophase

ⓔ **4/4 marks awarded** Student A has correctly recognised the stages of mitosis.

**(c)** The stain binds to the chromosomes, so they become visible.

ⓔ **1/1 mark awarded** Correct.

**(d)** This was to squash the root tip into a thin layer so that light could pass through the sample.

ⓔ **1/1 mark awarded** This answer makes an important point — an optical microscope depends on the specimen being thin enough to allow the transmission of light.

**(e)** $5\,mol\,dm^{-3}$ acid is highly concentrated and would be corrosive.

ⓔ **1/1 mark awarded** Student A has recognised that this concentration is very high and has correctly used the term 'corrosive'.

### Student B

**(a)** Nothing happens to the DNA during interphase. The cell is resting between divisions.

ⓔ **0/1 mark awarded** The idea that the cell is 'resting' during interphase is a common misconception. Although the cell is not dividing during interphase, the DNA is being replicated.

**(b)** B — metaphase, C — prophase, D — anaphase, E — telophase

ⓔ **2/4 marks awarded** Student B has mixed up anaphase and metaphase. Remember that the chromosomes line up in the **M**iddle of the cell during **M**etaphase and move **A**part during **A**naphase.

**(c)** So he could see the chromosomes.

ⓔ **1/1 mark awarded** This answer is not as detailed as student A's answer, but still gains the mark.

**(d)** To flatten the cells.

ⓔ **0/1 mark awarded** Pressing down on the coverslip would not squash individual cells, but would spread the cells out so they were in a single layer.

**(e)** The acid is very concentrated and could cause burns.

ⓔ **1/1 mark awarded** Although student B has not used the term 'corrosive', they have clearly suggested why the acid should be handled with caution.

# Question 3 The effect of sucrose concentration on osmosis

A student labelled six boiling tubes 0.0, 0.2, 0.4, 0.6, 0.8 and 1.0 mol dm$^{-3}$ sucrose solution. She used distilled water and a 1.0 mol dm$^{-3}$ sucrose solution to make up 20 cm$^3$ of each sucrose concentration in the boiling tubes. She then:

1   removed the 'skin' from a potato

2   cut six potato chips to the same length

3   weighed the chips and recorded their masses

4   put a chip into each boiling tube and left them for 30 minutes

5   gently blotted the potato chips dry

6   reweighed them and recorded their masses

7   repeated twice more to obtain three results for each concentration

She processed her results and found the percentage change in mass of the chip for each concentration. The student's results are shown in Table 1.

Table 1 The effect of sucrose concentration on the mass of potato tissue

| Concentration of sucrose solution/ mol dm$^{-3}$ | Initial mass/g | Final mass/g | Change in mass/g | Percentage change in mass | Mean percentage change in mass |
|---|---|---|---|---|---|
| 0.0 | 1.26 | 1.49 | 0.23 | 18.3 | 19.3 |
| | 1.26 | 1.51 | 0.25 | 19.8 | |
| | 1.22 | 1.46 | 0.24 | 19.7 | |
| 0.2 | 1.22 | 1.31 | 0.09 | 7.4 | 5.4 |
| | 1.27 | 1.32 | 0.05 | 3.9 | |
| | 1.25 | 1.31 | 0.06 | 4.8 | |
| 0.4 | 1.43 | 1.29 | −0.14 | −9.8 | −7.7 |
| | 1.32 | 1.26 | −0.06 | −4.5 | |
| | 1.37 | 1.25 | −0.12 | −8.8 | |
| 0.6 | 1.32 | 1.10 | −0.22 | −16.7 | −15.2 |
| | 1.26 | 1.07 | −0.19 | −15.1 | |
| | 1.22 | 1.05 | −0.17 | −13.9 | |
| 0.8 | 1.28 | 0.98 | −0.30 | −23.4 | −21.2 |
| | 1.25 | 1.01 | −0.24 | −19.2 | |
| | 1.23 | 0.97 | −0.26 | −21.1 | |
| 1.0 | 1.31 | 0.96 | −0.35 | −26.7 | −23.3 |
| | 1.27 | 1.00 | −0.27 | −21.3 | |
| | 1.23 | 0.96 | −0.27 | −22.0 | |

**(a)** Why did the student use potato chips from the same potato? (1 mark)

ⓔ Think of possible differences between cells from different potatoes.

**(b)** Describe how the student made $20\,cm^3$ of $0.6\,mol\,dm^{-3}$ sucrose solution. (1 mark)

ⓔ Although there is only 1 mark for the question, you need to state the volume of $1.0\,mol\,dm^{-3}$ sucrose solution used *and* the volume of distilled water.

**(c)** Suggest why the student removed the 'skin' from the potato. (1 mark)

ⓔ This is a 'suggest' question, which means you have to give a possible reason. In this question, you should consider how the 'skin', or the cells of the 'skin', might affect the investigation.

**(d)** Explain why the student processed her data to find the percentage change in mass. (1 mark)

ⓔ The key idea behind this question is that the potato cylinders did not have the same initial mass.

**(e)** Explain why the potato chip left in distilled water gained mass. (2 marks)

ⓔ Your answer needs to explain the direction of water movement in terms of osmosis and water potential.

**(f)** Describe how the student could use her processed data to find the water potential of the potato tissue. (3 marks)

ⓔ To answer this question, you need to describe how she would plot a graph, how she would determine the sucrose concentration of the potato tissue, and how she could then find the water potential.

---

**Student A**

**(a)** If the chips are from the same potato, all of the cells will have the same water potential.

---

ⓔ **1/1 mark awarded** Using the same potato means that the whole potato has been exposed to the same conditions before being cut into pieces.

---

**(b)** She used a measuring cylinder to measure out $12\,cm^3$ of $1.0\,mol\,dm^{-3}$ sucrose solution and poured it into a boiling tube. She then used a fresh measuring cylinder to measure $8\,cm^3$ of distilled water and poured this into the same boiling tube.

---

ⓔ **1/1 mark awarded** This is a detailed answer — only the volumes of solutions are required for the mark.

---

**(c)** The 'skin' is a different tissue from the rest of the potato and so would have a different water potential.

---

ⓔ **1/1 mark awarded** Student A gains the mark for stating that the 'skin' is a different tissue and for recognising that different tissues may have different water potentials.

**(d)** The initial mass of the potato chips was different, so working out the percentage change would allow her to make a valid comparison between the chips.

*e* **1/1 mark awarded** A correct and clear answer.

**(e)** The potato chips gained mass because water moved into the cells by osmosis. The water moved from a less negative $\psi$ outside the cells to a more negative $\psi$ inside the cells.

*e* **2/2 marks awarded** Student A has described the direction of water movement, stating that this was by osmosis, and correctly described the water potential as more negative inside the cells. The symbol $\psi$, representing water potential, is acceptable.

**(f)** The student should plot a graph with the sucrose concentration on the x-axis and the percentage change in mass on the y-axis. She should then find the point where the curve crosses the x-axis and read off the sucrose concentration. This concentration is the water potential of the potato tissue.

*e* **2/3 marks awarded** The description of how to plot and use the graph is clear, but the sucrose concentration of the tissue is not the same as its water potential. The water potential could be found using a table or graph showing the relationship between sucrose concentration and water potential. The point where the curve crosses the x-axis is known as the x-axis **intercept**.

## Student B

**(a)** So that the cells are genetically identical.

*e* **1/1 mark awarded** This is a different approach from student A's, but is an acceptable answer.

**(b)** She diluted 12 cm³ of sucrose solution with distilled water.

*e* **0/1 mark awarded** Student B needed to state the volume of distilled water as well as the volume of sucrose solution.

**(c)** The 'skin' might have a different water potential from the other cells.

*e* **0/1 mark awarded** Student B would have gained this marking point if they had said that the skin *cells* might have a different water potential.

**(d)** So she can compare potato chips with different starting masses.

*e* **1/1 mark awarded** This answer is not as detailed as the one above, but is enough to be awarded the mark.

(e) Water has moved into the cells from a high concentration to a low concentration.

*e* 0/2 marks awarded Although student B has correctly identified the direction of water movement, they have not used the terms *osmosis* or *water potential*, which are expected in an A-level answer.

(f) She should plot a graph of her results and find the concentration when there is no change in mass.

*e* 1/3 marks awarded Student B has been awarded a mark for stating how to use the graph, but more detail should have been included about how to plot the graph.

## Question 4 The effect of temperature on membrane permeability

A student carried out an investigation into the effect of temperature on the permeability of beetroot membranes. He:

1    cut ten discs of fresh beetroot and washed them thoroughly in distilled water.

2    collected five test tubes and measured $10\,cm^3$ of distilled water into each tube.

3    stood the test tubes in five separate water baths at 30, 40, 50, 60 and 70°C, and then left them for 5 minutes.

4    placed two beetroot discs in each tube and left them for 30 minutes, gently shaking the tubes every 5 minutes.

5    removed the beetroot discs after 30 minutes and poured each solution into a clean test tube.

6    used a colorimeter to measure the absorbance of each solution and then plotted a graph, as shown in Figure 3. The higher the absorbance, the more pigment has been released.

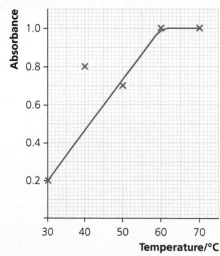

**Figure 3** Graph plotted by a student to show the effect of temperature on the permeability of beetroot membranes

**(a)** Why did the student wash the beetroot discs in distilled water after cutting them? (1 mark)

ⓔ Cutting the discs will damage the membranes of some of the beetroot cells, so you need to think about the effect this might have if the student did not wash the discs.

**(b)** Why were the test tubes of distilled water left in the water baths for 5 minutes before adding the beetroot? (1 mark)

ⓔ The distilled water measured into each tube would have been at room temperature, so your answer needs to explain what will happen to the temperature of the distilled water after 5 minutes in the water bath.

**(c)** Why did the student shake the test tubes every 5 minutes? (1 mark)

ⓔ When you are answering this question, your main consideration should be a factor that will affect the diffusion of the pigment out of the cells.

**(d)** Why did the student use fresh beetroot and not cooked beetroot? (1 mark)

ⓔ Cooked beetroot will have been exposed to high temperatures, so you need to consider the effect that this would have had on both the cell-surface membrane and the tonoplast.

**(e)** The student thinks that one of his results is anomalous. Describe what he should do. (2 marks)

ⓔ You may have been taught at GCSE to ignore anomalous results, but they should not be ignored. Think about the steps you would take if one of your results was anomalous.

**(f)** Describe the effect of increasing temperature on the permeability of the beetroot cell membranes. (2 marks)

ⓔ This is a 'describe' question, so you need to state the overall shape of the curve *and* use figures from the graph.

**(g)** Explain the shape of the curve between 60°C and 70°C. (1 mark)

ⓔ The curve reaches a plateau, or levels off, between these two temperatures. Your answer should give reasons why there is no further increase in absorbance by referring to the concentration of the pigment, or the damage to the membrane.

---

**Student A**

**(a)** This is so that any pigment in the distilled water has been released from the cells due to the effect of temperature on membrane permeability.

ⓔ **1/1 mark awarded** Correct — the cutting will have released pigment from damaged cells.

**(b)** This will allow the water to equilibrate.

ⓔ **1/1 mark awarded** This is a good term to use.

(c) This is to maintain the diffusion gradient for the pigment to pass out of the cells and into the distilled water.

**ⓔ 1/1 mark awarded** This is a good, clear answer.

(d) Cooking would involve the beetroot being heated to high temperatures that would denature the proteins in the plasma membranes and allow the pigment to leak out.

**ⓔ 1/1 mark awarded** This is a clear answer, which explains how cooking would affect the membrane proteins.

(e) He should repeat the experiment in exactly the same way.

**ⓔ 1/2 marks awarded** To gain the second mark, student A needed to state that the repeat is to check if the result is similar.

(f) There is a steady increase in permeability from 30°C to 60°C, then the curve reaches a plateau at an absorbance of 1.0.

**ⓔ 2/2 marks awarded** The overall shape of the curve has been clearly described and suitable values have been used to support this description.

(g) There is no further diffusion of pigment out of the cells because the concentration of pigment outside the cells is equal to the concentration inside the cells.

**ⓔ 1/1 mark awarded** This is a good answer, which gives a clear explanation in terms of diffusion and concentration.

### Student B

(a) This will remove any pigment from the surface of the discs.

**ⓔ 1/1 mark awarded** This is enough for the mark.

(b) So the water in each tube warms up to the required temperature.

**ⓔ 1/1 mark awarded** Although the term 'equilibrate' has not been used, student B is still awarded the mark for this explanation.

(c) Shaking the tube will stop the discs from sticking together, which would reduce the surface area for diffusion.

ⓔ **1/1 mark awarded** Although student B has not referred to the diffusion gradient, this is still a relevant comment that is worthy of the mark.

**(d)** Cooking beetroot would damage the membranes and the pigment would already have been released.

ⓔ **1/1 mark awarded** Although student B has not referred to denaturing of the proteins, they have been awarded a mark for the effect on the membrane and a mark for stating how this would affect the pigment.

**(e)** He should circle this result and ignore it when he is calculating his mean.

ⓔ **0/2 marks awarded** Anomalous results happen and should not be ignored.

**(f)** The permeability increases and then levels off.

ⓔ **1/2 marks awarded** Student B needed to include figures from the graph.

**(g)** All of the pigment has diffused out of the cells.

ⓔ **0/1 mark awarded** This answer is incorrect, but student B could have written that the pigment was diffusing in and out of the cells at the same rate.

## Question 5 Estimating the number of stomata

A student observed the structures involved in gas exchange in a leaf. He removed a small piece of the lower epidermis and viewed it using an optical microscope. He counted the number of stomata that he could see in the field of view and used this to estimate the total number of stomata present in the lower epidermis of the leaf. Figure 4 shows the lower epidermis as viewed by the student.

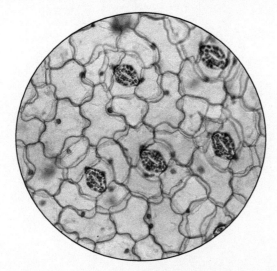

**Figure 4** Stomata in the lower epidermis of a leaf, as seen using an optical microscope

**(a)** Describe how the student could prepare a piece of the lower epidermis to observe using an optical microscope. (3 marks)

ⓔ This question requires you to describe the method you would use to prepare a slide. Your answer should be logical and include the terms 'slide' and 'coverslip'.

**(b)** The student used an optical microscope with an eyepiece lens magnification of ×10 and objective lenses of ×4, ×10 and ×40. Calculate the maximum magnification that the student used. (1 mark)

ⓔ Magnification is calculated using both the eyepiece and the objective lens.

**(c)** Describe how the student could have used a clear ruler with mm divisions to find the area of the field of view using the low-power objective lens. (2 marks)

ⓔ The field of view refers to the circle that you can see when you look down an optical microscope. One of the maths skills that you may be assessed on is your ability to calculate the area of a circle. You will need to state the measurement you will take and then how you will use this to calculate area.

**(d)** The student found that there were five stomata per mm². Describe how he could have estimated the total number of stomata in the lower epidermis of one leaf. (3 marks)

ⓔ To answer this question, you firstly need to describe how you would find the area of the leaf. You then need to use the number of stomata given to describe how you would estimate the total number of stomata.

---

**Student A**

**(a)** He should take a clean glass slide and add one drop of water to the centre of the slide. He then needs to peel off the lower epidermis, which is thin as it is a single layer of cells, and lay it on the slide. Finally, he should cover the epidermis with a coverslip.

---

ⓔ **2/3 marks awarded** This is a well-structured answer, but needs more detail in the final sentence to minimise the risk of trapping air bubbles — for example, position the coverslip on the slide at an angle of 45° to the specimen and then gently lower it onto the slide using a mounted needle.

**(b)** total magnification = eyepiece lens × objective lens = 10 × 40 = ×400

ⓔ **1/1 mark awarded** It is always a good idea to show your working.

**(c)** He could put the ruler on the stage and focus on the scale, then measure the diameter of the field of view. He can then use $\pi r^2$ to calculate the area of the field of view.

ⓔ **2/2 marks awarded** This is a good answer that describes both steps clearly.

**(d)** He could use a piece of squared paper to draw round the leaf. Then he could count the number of squares to find the total area of the leaf in $mm^2$. He knows that there are five stomata in each $mm^2$, so he can multiply the area of the leaf by 5.

*e* **3/3 marks awarded** This is a concise, clear answer.

**Student B**

**(a)** The leaf should be put on a glass slide with a drop of water, then a coverslip put over it.

*e* **1/3 marks awarded** Student B understands the overall process, but this answer omits two important steps: the plant tissue must be thin, so just a piece of lower epidermis should be used and not the whole leaf; the method must avoid trapping air bubbles.

**(b)** ×400

*e* **1/1 mark awarded** The mark is awarded for the correct answer.

**(c)** He could look at the ruler down the microscope and measure the width of the field of view and then use this to find its area.

*e* **1/2 marks awarded** Student B needed to describe how to find the area by stating the equation.

**(d)** Find the area of the leaf in $mm^2$, then times by 5 to get total number of stomata.

*e* **2/3 marks awarded** Student B needed to describe *how* the area of the leaf could be found.

# Question 6 The effect of antibiotics on bacterial growth

A student investigated the effect of antibiotics on the growth of bacteria. She used aseptic techniques to:

1  transfer $1\,cm^3$ of liquid bacterial culture to an agar plate

2  spread the bacterial culture to cover the plate

3  place four paper discs soaked in antibiotic on the plate

The student incubated the agar plate at 25°C for 48 hours. Figure 5 shows the appearance of the plate following incubation.

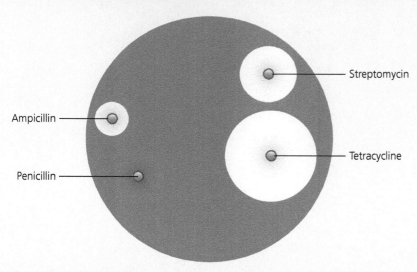

**Figure 5** A diagram to show the appearance of an agar plate with antibiotic discs following incubation

**(a)** Describe *two* aseptic techniques that the student could have used. (2 marks)

ⓔ You are expected to have used aseptic techniques to minimise contamination and should be able to describe some of the methods that you used.

**(b)** Give *one* reason why the student used aseptic technique. (1 mark)

ⓔ Be specific when answering this question and avoid vague references to bacteria escaping.

**(c)** The student incubated the agar plates at 25°C. Suggest *one* reason why she did not incubate them at a higher temperature. (1 mark)

ⓔ A higher temperature would be closer to human body temperature. Your answer needs to give a possible reason for the student using a lower temperature.

The student measured the diameter of the clear zone around each antibiotic and recorded the results in Table 2.

**Table 2** The diameter of clear zones around antibiotic discs

| Antibiotic | Mean diameter of the clear zone/mm |
|------------|-----------------------------------|
| Ampicillin | 9 |
| Streptomycin | 15 |
| Tetracycline | 24 |
| Penicillin | 0 |

**(d)** Calculate the area of the clear zone around tetracycline. Use π = 3.14. (1 mark)

ⓔ Calculating the area of a circle is one of the maths skills named in the specification. You are expected to know the formula.

**(e)** The student concluded that penicillin was not effective against this bacterium. Explain why she reached this conclusion. (1 mark)

*e* Your answer should not just be a statement that there is no clear zone; it should include an explanation *why*.

### Student A

**(a)** Use a sterile pipette to transfer the bacterial culture to the agar plate. Flame the neck of the bottle containing the bacterial culture.

*e* **2/2 marks awarded** These are two clearly described techniques that show student A's familiarity with the practical.

**(b)** This technique minimises the risk of bacteria from the air contaminating the agar plate.

*e* **1/1 mark awarded** This is a well-expressed answer, with good use of the term 'contaminating'.

**(c)** A higher temperature could be closer to the optimum temperature for bacteria that cause human disease. This would be dangerous for the student.

*e* **1/1 mark awarded** This is exactly why the incubation temperature should not exceed 25°C.

**(d)** Diameter of clear zone for tetracycline = 24 mm, so radius = 12 mm.
area of clear zone = $\pi r^2$ = 3.14 × $12^2$ = 452.16 mm$^2$

*e* **1/1 mark awarded** Although the mark would be awarded for giving the correct answer, it is good practice to show your working in this way.

**(e)** There is no clear zone around the penicillin, so this antibiotic did not inhibit the growth of the bacteria.

*e* **1/1 mark awarded** Another well-written answer, with good use of the term 'inhibit'.

### Student B

**(a)** Work next to a lit Bunsen burner. Wash hands thoroughly before and after the practical.

*e* **1/2 marks awarded** Student B's first point is specific to microbial aseptic technique, but hand washing is an example of good practice that relates to all practical activities. A better answer could refer to wiping down the bench with disinfectant before and after the practical.

(b) These techniques protect the student from harmful bacteria.

ⓔ 0/1 mark awarded This answer is too vague to gain the mark. A more specific answer might say 'these techniques prevent the release of harmful bacteria into the air'.

(c) This is the optimum temperature for bacteria, so they will grow better.

ⓔ 0/1 mark awarded Although this may be the optimum temperature for some bacteria, this answer does not reflect the understanding expected at A-level.

(d) 75.36 mm$^2$

ⓔ 0/1 mark awarded This is an incorrect answer because student B did not use the correct formula. They have used $\pi d$, which is the formula for the circumference of a circle, and have not shown any working.

(e) The bacteria could grow next to this antibiotic, showing that penicillin did not kill the bacteria or slow their growth.

ⓔ 1/1 mark awarded This is a simply expressed answer, but it shows understanding of the practical results and gains the mark.

# Question 7 Using chromatography to investigate leaf pigments

A student investigated the pigments present in two different leaves, A and B. The steps he followed were:

1 Crush each leaf with solvent to extract the pigments.

2 Label two strips of filter paper A and B.

3 Draw a pencil line 1 cm from the bottom of each strip of paper.

4 Use a fine glass tube to put a spot of extract from leaf A on the pencil line on paper A.

5 Put a spot of extract from leaf B on the pencil line on paper B.

6 Stand each strip of filter paper in a boiling tube of solvent; check that the solvent is not above the pencil line.

7 Leave the strips of filter paper in the boiling tubes for 30 minutes without moving them.

8 Remove each strip of filter paper and draw a pencil line to show how far the solvent has travelled.

Figure 6 shows the appearance of one of the completed chromatograms.

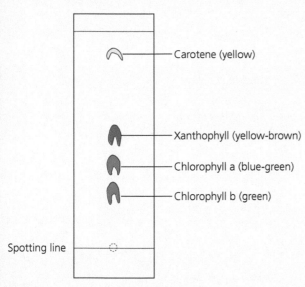

**Figure 6** Plant pigments separated on a paper chromatogram

**(a)** Explain why the student used pencil to draw the spotting line and not pen. (1 mark)

ⓔ When answering this question, remember that the ink used in pens might be soluble in the solvent you are using.

**(b)** Explain why the student checked that the solvent in the boiling tube was not above the pencil line. (1 mark)

ⓔ The pigment spot is on the pencil line, so you need to describe what would happen to the pigment if the solvent were above it.

**(c)** Suggest why the student did not move the boiling tubes once the filter paper was inside. (1 mark)

ⓔ Moving the boiling tubes will move the solvent in the bottom of the tubes. Your answer needs to describe how the solution not being level might affect the movement of either the solvent or the pigments.

**(d)** Explain why the student drew a line to show how far the solvent travelled as soon as he removed it from the tube. (1 mark)

ⓔ You need to know how far the solvent has travelled to calculate the Rf value. You need to think about what will happen to the solvent on the filter paper once it has been removed from the tube.

**(e)** The student wants to calculate the Rf value of a pigment so he can compare his results with those of another student. Describe how he would calculate the Rf value of a pigment. (2 marks)

ⓔ Look at the number of marks available for this question. You need to state the measurements that you would need to make and how you would use these measurements.

**Student A**

**(a)** Pencil would not dissolve in the solvent.

*e* **1/1 mark awarded** This is a clear and concise answer that gains the mark.

**(b)** The pigments found from the leaves are soluble in the solvent and would be removed from the paper if the solvent were above the pencil line.

*e* **1/1 mark awarded** This answer makes good use of the terms 'soluble' and 'solvent'.

**(c)** Moving the tubes would move the solvent in the bottom of the tube and might cause it to travel up the paper at an angle instead of running straight.

*e* **1/1 mark awarded** This is a good point — the solvent travelling at an angle might affect the movement of the pigment and the calculation of Rf values.

**(d)** The solvent would evaporate and you would not be able to see the solvent front.

*e* **1/1 mark awarded** Good use of the term 'solvent front' — this term was not used in the question to describe the distance travelled by the solvent.

**(e)** He should measure the distance from the origin to the centre of the pigment spot and measure the distance from the origin to the solvent front. The Rf value is calculated using distance travelled by pigment divided by distance travelled by solvent.

*e* **2/2 marks awarded** Measuring to the centre of the pigment spot is an excellent way of standardising the procedure, but the answer would still have gained full marks without this point. Good use of terminology again: for example, 'origin' was not used in the question to describe the pencil line.

**Student B**

**(a)** The pen might travel up the filter paper.

*e* **0/1 mark awarded** Student B has an idea of what might happen, but this is poorly expressed and no mark is awarded. A better answer might say 'the ink from the pen might run with the solvent'.

**(b)** If the solvent was above the pencil line it might wash the pigments off.

ⓔ **1/1 mark awarded** This is a basic answer, but is worth 1 mark despite the simple terms used.

> **(c)** The pigments might run off the side of the paper.

ⓔ **1/1 mark awarded** This is another basic answer that just gains the mark.

> **(d)** The paper will dry quickly and you will not be able to see how far the solvent travelled.

ⓔ **1/1 mark awarded** Student B has not used the terms 'evaporate' or 'solvent front', but has included the key idea and gained the mark.

> **(e)** The distance travelled by the solvent is divided by the distance travelled by the pigment.

ⓔ **1/2 marks awarded** A mark is awarded here for the implication that these distances have to be measured, but student B has the measurements the wrong way round.

## Question 8 Investigating photosynthesis using a chloroplast suspension

A student carried out an investigation using a chloroplast suspension and a blue dye called DCPIP. When DCPIP is reduced, it changes colour from blue to colourless. The student made a suspension of chloroplasts by blending leaves with ice-cold isolation medium and then filtering. She set up three boiling tubes, as shown in Table 3, covered tube 2 with foil, and then stood all three tubes next to a bright light for 2 hours. Table 3 shows the contents of each tube and its appearance at the beginning and end of the investigation.

**Table 3** The effect of a chloroplast suspension on the colour of DCPIP

| Tube number | Contents of the tube | Appearance at the start of the investigation | Appearance after 2 hours |
|---|---|---|---|
| 1 | Chloroplast suspension Buffer at pH 7 DCPIP | Blue | Green |
| 2 | Chloroplast suspension Buffer at pH 7 DCPIP | Blue | Blue |
| 3 | Boiled chloroplast suspension Buffer at pH 7 DCPIP | Blue | Blue |

**(a)** Explain the colour change in tube 1. (2 marks)

ⓔ The DCPIP has been decolourised, meaning that the DCPIP has been reduced. You need to use your knowledge of chlorophyll and the electron transfer chain to explain how DCPIP was reduced.

**(b)** The student covered tube 2 with foil. Explain why the DCPIP in this tube remained blue. (2 marks)

ⓔ DCPIP will decolourise when it accepts electrons. Your answer needs to demonstrate your understanding of the transfer of electrons during photosynthesis.

**(c)** Explain why the student used isolation medium that was ice-cold. (2 marks)

ⓔ Blending the leaves will break open the leaf cells, releasing the cell contents, including enzymes. Your answer needs to make the link between enzyme activity and the isolation medium being ice-cold.

**(d)** The isolation medium contained sucrose. Explain why sucrose was included in the isolation medium. (2 marks)

ⓔ Your answer needs you to explain what would happen if the chloroplasts were in water rather than in a sucrose solution. How would chloroplasts be affected by water entering or leaving them?

**(e)** Explain why the DCPIP in tube 3 did not decolourise. (2 marks)

ⓔ The chloroplast suspension in tube 3 had been boiled. Your answer needs to include the effect of boiling on proteins and how this would affect photosynthesis.

---

**Student A**

**(a)** The DCPIP has decolourised so has been reduced. This means that DCPIP has accepted electrons released from chlorophyll that have been transferred along the electron transfer chain.

ⓔ **2/2 marks awarded** Student A has gained marks here for their understanding of the decolourisation of DCPIP and for explaining the movement of electrons.

**(b)** The foil prevented light from reaching the chlorophyll, so photoionisation did not take place and no electrons were released from the chlorophyll molecule. This meant that no electrons were available to reduce DCPIP, so it stayed blue.

ⓔ **2/2 marks awarded** This is a detailed, well-written answer that demonstrates a good understanding of the role of light in photosynthesis.

**(c)** Blending the leaves releases enzymes from the cell that could damage the chloroplasts. An ice-cold buffer will reduce the rate of enzyme activity and prevent chloroplast damage.

---

**ⓔ 2/2 marks awarded** Releasing enzymes such as lipases and proteases, which are normally compartmentalised within lysosomes, could lead to the breakdown of the chloroplast membranes. Reducing the activity of these enzymes is essential for the chloroplasts to continue functioning.

**(d)** The presence of sucrose reduced the water potential of the isolation medium. This meant that there was no net movement of water into the chloroplasts. If water entered the chloroplasts by osmosis, they would burst.

**ⓔ 2/2 marks awarded** This is an excellent answer that shows clear understanding of the term 'water potential' and relates this to an effect on the chloroplasts.

**(e)** Boiling would denature the proteins in the chloroplasts, including those that make up the electron transfer chain. Electrons would not pass along the electron transfer chain and so cannot be accepted by DCPIP.

**ⓔ 2/2 marks awarded** The first mark is awarded for explaining that the proteins in the electron transfer chain are denatured, and the second mark for explaining why this would prevent the reduction of DCPIP.

### Student B

**(a)** The DCPIP has lost its blue colour. This means that it has been reduced, so has gained electrons.

**ⓔ 0/2 marks awarded** Stating that DCPIP changes colour when it is reduced is just repeating the stem of the question, so no mark is awarded for this. Student B knows that reduction is gain of electrons, but this is not worthy of a mark at A-level. Some reference to chlorophyll as the source of the electrons should have been made.

**(b)** The foil blocks out light, so no photosynthesis can occur.

**ⓔ 0/2 marks awarded** Although student B makes the link between blocking out light and photosynthesis, this answer lacks the necessary details and terminology that student A includes in their answer.

**(c)** This will reduce the kinetic energy of the enzymes, so chemical reactions will happen more slowly.

**ⓔ 1/2 marks awarded** A mark is awarded for recognising that the low temperature will reduce the rate of enzyme activity, but this needs to be linked to an effect on the chloroplasts.

(d) Having sucrose in the isolation medium means that no osmosis will take place, so no water will move into or out of the cell. If water moved into the cells by osmosis, the cells might burst.

ⓔ 0/2 marks awarded Although student B recognises that the presence of sucrose has an effect on osmosis, there is no reference to water potential and saying that there is 'no osmosis' is poor phrasing. This answer does not gain the second mark because student B refers to cells bursting rather than describing the effect on chloroplasts; the leaf cells have already been ruptured by blending, and plant cells would not burst anyway due to their cell walls.

(e) The chloroplast suspension was boiled in tube 3 and proteins are denatured at high temperatures. The light-dependent reaction of photosynthesis would not take place.

ⓔ 1/2 marks awarded This answer is awarded 1 mark for correctly describing the effect of temperature on proteins, but student B has not fully answered the question because they have not explained why this would prevent the reduction of DCPIP.

## Question 9 Using a respirometer to investigate oxygen uptake

A student put 2 g of yeast into a glucose solution. He used the apparatus shown in Figure 7 to investigate the rate of oxygen uptake by the culture of yeast at 30°C.

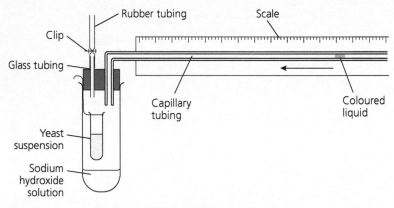

**Figure 7** A simple respirometer

(a) The drop of coloured liquid moves through the capillary tubing towards the yeast suspension (as shown by the arrow in Figure 7). Explain why the liquid moves in the direction shown. (3 marks)

ⓔ This question is about pressure differences. The yeast is respiring aerobically and so is taking in oxygen and releasing carbon dioxide. The carbon dioxide is absorbed by the sodium hydroxide. How would this affect the pressure inside the tube compared with outside the tube?

The student recorded the volume at the start of his investigation and took a reading from the scale every 10 minutes. His results are shown in Table 4.

**Table 4** Volume readings from a respirometer taken at 10-minute intervals

| Time/min | Volume reading on the scale/cm$^3$ |
|----------|-----------------------------------|
| 0 | 3.2 |
| 10 | 3.8 |
| 20 | 4.5 |
| 30 | 5.0 |
| 40 | 5.4 |
| 50 | 5.6 |
| 60 | 5.7 |

**(b)** Plot a graph of these results. (A grid will be provided in the exam paper.)　　(5 marks)

ⓔ Marks may be available for having the axes the correct way round, choosing a suitable scale, labelling the axes, accurately plotting points and drawing a suitable line.

**(c)** Calculate the rate of oxygen use per gram of yeast during this investigation. Include a suitable unit.　　(2 marks)

ⓔ You need to use two numbers to calculate the rate: the volume of oxygen taken up in 1 hour and the mass of yeast.

**(d)** The student repeated the investigation at 20°C and found that the volume of oxygen taken up by the yeast was lower. Explain why.　　(1 mark)

ⓔ This question requires you to apply your knowledge and make the link between temperature and respiration.

---

**Student A**

**(a)** The yeast respires aerobically, taking in oxygen and releasing carbon dioxide. Carbon dioxide is absorbed by potassium hydroxide decreasing the pressure inside the tube so that it is less than atmospheric pressure and the liquid moves to the left (as shown by the arrow).

---

ⓔ **3/3 marks awarded** The marks are awarded for stating that oxygen is taken in, and that carbon dioxide is absorbed, and for explaining how this affects pressure.

**(b)**

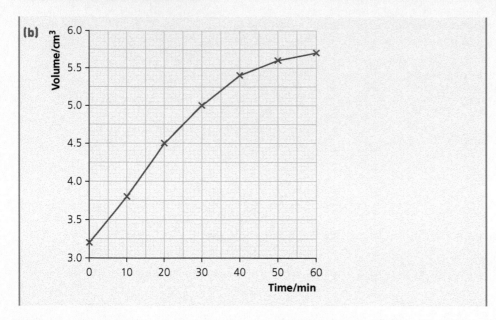

**ⓔ 5/5 marks awarded** The axes are the correct way round, with the IV on the x-axis; a suitable scale has been chosen, making good use of the grid; axes are fully labelled and units included; points are plotted clearly and correctly; a suitable line has been drawn.

**(c)** rate of oxygen use = 5.7 – 3.2 = 2.5 cm³ in 1 hour
There are 2 g of yeast, so oxygen use = 1.25 cm³ g⁻¹ hour⁻¹.

**ⓔ 2/2 marks awarded** Working has been clearly shown and a suitable unit chosen. The rate could also be given per minute: 1.25/60 = 0.02 cm³ min⁻¹ g⁻¹.

**(d)** The rate of respiration is higher at 30°C because this is closer to the optimum temperature for the enzymes involved in respiration.

**ⓔ 1/1 mark awarded** This is an excellent answer, with good use of scientific terminology.

## Student B

**(a)** The liquid moves because the carbon dioxide produced by respiration is absorbed by the potassium hydroxide, creating a vacuum that sucks the liquid along the tube.

**ⓔ 1/3 marks awarded** Student B has been awarded a mark for stating that the carbon dioxide has been absorbed, but there is no reference to oxygen uptake or the effect on pressure. The term 'vacuum' is incorrect and 'sucks the liquid along' is a poor expression.

**(b)**

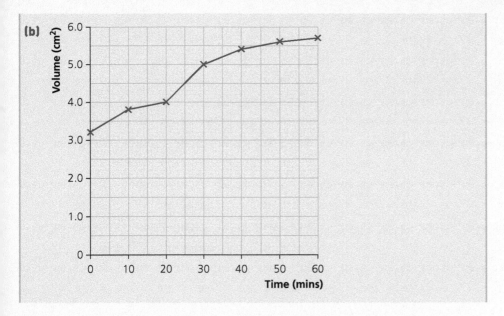

**ⓔ 2/5 marks awarded** The axes are the correct way round and a suitable scale has been chosen, but the $y$-axis scale means that there is a lot of unused space. Marks have been lost because the point at 20 minutes has been plotted incorrectly and the wrong unit has been used on the $y$-axis ($cm^2$ instead of $cm^3$). The units should have a solidus before them rather than being written in brackets, but you would not be penalised marks for writing them in this format.

**(c)** 2 g of yeast takes up $2.5\,cm^3$ of oxygen in 60 minutes, so 1 g of yeast takes up $0.02\,cm^3$ of oxygen in 1 minute.

**ⓔ 1/2 marks awarded** Student B shows a good understanding of the data and this is a clearly presented calculation, but the unit for rate has not been written correctly as $cm^3\,min^{-1}\,g^{-1}$.

**(d)** Less oxygen is taken up because the yeast is respiring less.

**ⓔ 0/1 mark awarded** This is insufficient for a mark because there is no explanation of *why* the rate of respiration is lower.

## Question 10 The effect of light on maggot behaviour

A student investigated the effect of light on the behaviour of maggots using a choice chamber. She put damp filter paper in the bottom of the choice chamber, then covered half of the chamber with light-proof black cloth and left the other half uncovered (Figure 8). Using a small plastic spoon, she added 12 maggots to the chamber and left them for 10 minutes. She recorded the number of maggots in each half of the choice chamber every minute for 10 minutes.

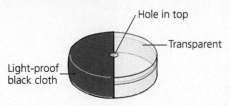

**Figure 8** A diagram to show how the student set up the choice chamber

**(a)** Suggest why the student put damp filter paper in each half of the choice chamber. (1 mark)

ⓔ Your answer should focus on the environmental conditions, while writing in an appropriate scientific style.

**(b)** Suggest why the student used a plastic spoon to pick up the maggots and not a pair of forceps. (1 mark)

ⓔ The ethical use of organisms is one of the skills you are expected to have developed, so your answer should consider the effect on the animals.

**Table 5** Mean number of maggots present in each half of the choice chamber

| Environmental condition | Mean number of maggots present per minute |
|---|---|
| Dark | 10 |
| Light | 2 |

**(c)** Table 5 shows that more maggots were recorded in dark conditions than light. Explain why this behaviour would be an advantage to maggots. (1 mark)

ⓔ Your answer should be specific and should indicate how this response to light would increase the organism's chance of survival.

**(d)** The student wanted to determine whether there was a significant difference between her observed and expected results.

   **(i)** State a null hypothesis for the student's investigation. (1 mark)

ⓔ Remember that a null hypothesis is a testable statement that there would be no difference.

   **(ii)** Use the null hypothesis to state the expected number of maggots in each area of the choice chamber after 10 minutes. (1 mark)

ⓔ Refer to your null hypothesis from part (i) and the total number of maggots given in the question.

   **(iii)** State the statistical test that the student should use to analyse her results. Give the reason for your choice of test. (2 marks)

ⓔ The first mark is for simply stating the name of the statistical test. The second mark is for giving your reason. The maths skills section for required practical 10 gives information about the three statistical tests you need to know and when they should be used.

**Student A**

**(a)** Damp conditions provide a more favourable environment for maggots as this prevents them from drying out.

ⓔ **1/1 mark awarded** This is a good, concise answer.

**(b)** She might squeeze a pair of forceps too hard and harm the maggots.

ⓔ **1/1 mark awarded** This is a simple example of the ethical use of animals.

**(c)** If the maggots move towards dark regions, they are less likely to be seen by predators and this increases their chance of survival.

ⓔ **1/1 mark awarded** It also encourages them to burrow into their food and avoid drying out.

**(d) (i)** There is no difference in the number of maggots found in light and dark conditions.

ⓔ **1/1 mark awarded** This is a concise null hypothesis.

**(ii)** There would be six maggots in each half.

ⓔ **1/1 mark awarded** In other words, the 12 maggots divided equally between each half.

**(iii)** She needs to use the chi-squared test because the data are categoric and she is comparing the frequencies.

ⓔ **2/2 marks awarded** This is a good explanation for the choice of statistical test. Student A has also correctly used the word 'data' as a plural (data *are* categoric, not data *is* categoric).

**Student B**

**(a)** This is because maggots like damp conditions.

ⓔ 0/1 mark awarded Avoid attributing human feelings and emotions to simple animals. The maggots do not 'like' damp conditions, but it is their preferred environment.

(b) The maggots might get stressed if they were picked up using forceps.

ⓔ 0/1 mark awarded Describing maggots as 'stressed' is poor biology and not worthy of a mark at A-level.

(c) The maggots are trying to avoid predators by hiding in the dark.

ⓔ 0/1 mark awarded This is another example of poor biology, with the suggestion that maggots are intentionally moving to the darker environment to avoid predation.

(d) (i) There is no significant difference between the results.

ⓔ 0/1 mark awarded This is too vague and makes no reference to the different conditions.

(ii) I would expect most of the maggots to be in the dark.

ⓔ 0/1 mark awarded The question relates to a statistical test, so the term 'expected' should be used in that context rather than interpreted as what you expect to happen.

(iii) The stats test she should use is the chi-squared test because she is comparing observed and expected results.

ⓔ 1/2 marks awarded Only the mark for the choice of test has been awarded because the reason for the choice is too vague. Student B should have referred to the type of data — categoric.

# Question 11 Using a calibration curve to find glucose concentration

A student was given glucose solutions of concentrations 2, 4, 6, 8 and 10%. The method followed by the student is given below:

1  Add dilute sulfuric acid and a solution of potassium manganate(VII) to each glucose concentration.

2  Time how long each concentration takes to change colour from pink to colourless.

3  Repeat steps 1 and 2 for each concentration.

4  Plot a graph of the results (Figure 9).

5  Use this graph to estimate the concentration of an unknown glucose solution.

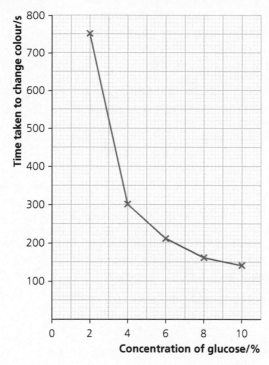

**Figure 9** Graph of time taken to change colour against glucose concentration

**(a)** The student had to decide when the pink colour had completely disappeared. Suggest how he ensured that his decision was consistent. (1 mark)

ⓔ There are different ways of approaching this question, but your answer could include a colour comparison.

**(b)** Explain why the student repeated steps 1 and 2 for each concentration. (1 mark)

ⓔ This question asks you to *explain*, so you need to make sure that your answer includes enough detail — 'to calculate the mean' would be insufficient.

**(c)** The student estimated the concentration of the unknown solution to be 5%. Explain why this was only an estimate. (1 mark)

ⓔ The points on the graph have been joined, because the student could not be certain of the intermediate values. Your answer should refer to concentrations that have not been tested.

**(d)** Explain how the student could modify his method to find a more accurate concentration of the unknown solution. (1 mark)

ⓔ The method should be modified to include more concentrations of glucose, but your answer should specify the range of concentrations.

> **Student A**
>
> **(a)** He could use a solution that had already completely decolourised, and then compare all of the other solutions with this one.

**ⓔ 1/1 mark awarded** This technique is called using a colour standard and would allow a consistent end-point to be determined.

**(b)** This was so he could show that his measurements were repeatable and could identify any anomalous results.

**ⓔ 1/1 mark awarded** The word 'repeatable' is used well here because the student repeated the experiment using the same equipment and method. Measurements would be **reproducible** if another person carried out the investigation and obtained the same results.

**(c)** It is only an estimate because the student did not test a 5% glucose concentration.

**ⓔ 1/1 mark awarded** This concise answer gains the mark.

**(d)** He should repeat the experiment, but using more concentrations between 4 and 6%, for example 4.5, 5.0 and 5.5%.

**ⓔ 1/1 mark awarded** This detailed answer would still gain the mark for just stating 'values between 4 and 6%' without specifying the concentrations.

## Student B

**(a)** He could put a piece of white card behind each solution to check that there is no pink colour left.

**ⓔ 1/1 mark awarded** This answer is more simply expressed than student A's, but is still worthy of a mark.

**(b)** Having repeats allows you to identify anomalous results. These can be ignored when you are calculating the mean.

**ⓔ 0/1 mark awarded** Anomalous results should not be ignored — possible reasons for the anomaly should be investigated.

**(c)** The student did not test the intermediate values between 4 and 6%.

**ⓔ 1/1 mark awarded** This answer is phrased slightly differently from student A's response, but still gains the mark.

**(d)** He should test more concentrations around 5%.

🅔 **1/1 mark awarded** Although student B has not suggested specific concentrations, 'around 5%' gives enough information to gain the mark.

# Question 12 The effect of distance from a tree on leaf size

A student investigated the effect of distance from a tree on leaf shape and size. She measured the length of dandelion leaves at different distances from a tree and counted the number of lobes present on each leaf (Figure 10).

**(a)**  **(b)**

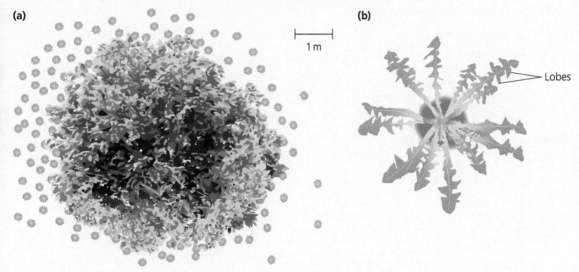

**Figure 10** (a) A tree surrounded by dandelion plants, as viewed from above.
(b) A dandelion plant as viewed from above, showing leaf lobes

**(a) (i)**  Name an environmental variable that could affect leaf length. (1 mark)

🅔 You could name any biotic or abiotic factor that could realistically have an effect on the size of leaves.

**(ii)** Explain how the variable named in (i) could affect leaf length. (1 mark)

🅔 Make sure that your answer is linked to the variable you gave in (i) and describes its effect on a biological process related to leaf size, such as photosynthesis or respiration.

**(b)**  The student measured the length of the dandelion leaves. Give *one* reason why leaf length may not be the best way to measure leaf size. (1 mark)

🅔 You just need to give the name of one other measure of leaf size that could vary.

**(c)**  Suggest *one* reason why the student measured the leaves while they were still attached to the plant. (1 marks)

🅔 Your answer could refer to an ethical reason for not removing the leaves, or to the effect removing the leaves would have on the measurements.

**(d)** The student plotted a graph of distance from the base of the tree in metres against the mean dandelion leaf length in mm.

Describe how the student could have used a quadrat and tape measure to collect the data for this graph. (2 marks)

🄴 To plot the graph, the student would have to measure the length of leaves at specific distances from the tree, so your answer should describe the use of a belt transect. This is *not* random sampling.

The student plotted a graph of leaf length against the number of lobes per leaf and concluded that there was a positive correlation.

**(e) (i)** Name the type of graph that the student should have plotted. Give a reason for your answer. (1 mark)

🄴 Notice that you need to name the type of graph *and* explain your choice of graph. Make sure that you give a specific reason related to the type of data collected.

**(ii)** What does *positive correlation* mean? (1 mark)

🄴 This is a straightforward recall question, assessing your understanding of this term.

> **Student A**
>
> **(a) (i)** light intensity

🄴 **1/1 mark awarded** Student A has correctly identified a factor that could affect leaf size.

> **(ii)** Light intensity would affect the rate of photosynthesis, which may affect leaf length.

🄴 **1/1 mark awarded** A clear link has been made to photosynthesis.

> **(b)** Leaves might be different widths as well as different lengths.

🄴 **1/1 mark awarded** Student A recognises that length is not the only measurement of leaf size.

> **(c)** Picking the leaves might damage the plant. The leaves might dry out and shrink once they have been picked, which would reduce their size.

🄴 **1/1 mark awarded** Student A has included two acceptable points here, but only 1 mark is available.

**(d)** To collect these data, she would have laid the tape measure out perpendicular to the tree and positioned the quadrat at regular intervals, about every 2m. She would then measure the length of the leaves and find the mean leaf length.

*e* **2/2 marks awarded** The technique is clearly described, with the correct uses of both the tape measure and the quadrat.

**(e) (i)** She should draw a scatter graph because she is looking for a relationship between two continuous variables.

*e* **1/1 mark awarded** This is a good answer that names the type of graph and gives a clear reason for the choice.

**(ii)** Positive correlation means that as one variable increases, so does the other variable.

*e* **1/1 mark awarded** Student A's answer gains the mark for a general explanation of the term.

**Student B**

**(a) (i)** temperature

*e* **1/1 mark awarded** This is another abiotic factor that would affect leaf size. Examples of biotic factors could be predation or disease.

**(ii)** Respiration involves a series of enzyme-controlled reactions, so it would be affected by temperature. Less respiration might lead to less leaf growth.

*e* **1/1 mark awarded** The mark has been awarded for linking temperature to respiration, but it would be better to say 'a reduced rate of respiration' than 'less respiration'.

**(b)** Some leaves might be wider or thicker.

*e* **1/1 mark awarded** This is a good point, especially the reference to variation in leaf thickness.

**(c)** Picking the leaves harms the environment, and she might mix up the leaves and forget where she picked them.

*e* **0/1 mark awarded** Neither of these points is worthy of a mark. The term 'environment' is too vague, whereas referring to damage to the *habitat* or *ecosystem* would gain a mark. References to human error that suggest poor experimental technique would not be credited at A-level.

(d) She would have used the tape measure to map out a grid and used the quadrat to take random samples.

*e* 0/2 marks awarded Student B has described a random sampling technique that is not appropriate for this investigation.

(e) (i) The student should have drawn a scattergram because she is looking for a relationship between pairs of measurements.

*e* 1/1 mark awarded Scattergram, scatter graph and scatter diagram are all terms that could be used to describe this type of graph. Although student B has not included the term 'continuous' when describing the variables, they still gain a mark for stating that the measurements are in pairs.

(ii) This means that as the length of the leaf increases, the number of lobes also increases.

*e* 1/1 mark awarded Student B has linked the answer to the example given and gains the mark.

# Index